VI
information

What you need to know
A B O U T
Perimenopause

BY BERNARD J. CORTESE, M.D.

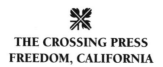

THE CROSSING PRESS
FREEDOM, CALIFORNIA

Dedicated to us, the "Baby Boomers,"
as we celebrate our journey through life.

Copyright © 1998 by Bernard J. Cortese
Cover design by Victoria May
Interior design by Magnolia Studio
Printed in the U.S.A.

The information contained in this book is not intended as a substitute for consulting your physician or other health care provider. Any attempt to diagnose and treat an illness should be done under the direction of a health care professional. The publisher does not advocate the use of any particular health care protocol, but believes that the information in this book should be available to the public. The publisher and author are not responsible for any adverse effects or consequences resulting from the use of any of the suggestions, preparations, or procedures discussed in this book.

For information on bulk purchases or group discounts for this and other Crossing Press titles, please contact our Special Sales Manager at 800-777-1048.

Visit our Web site on the Internet: www.crossingpress.com

Library of Congress Cataloging-in-Publication Data
Cortese, Bernard.
     Perimenopause / by Bernard Cortese.
        p. cm. (Vital information series)
     Includes index.
     ISBN 0-89594-914-8 (pbk.)
     1. Perimenopause--Popular works. I. Title.
RG188.C67   1998
618.1'75--dc21   98-26905
                                        CIP

Contents

Introduction

Perimenopause is the word that refers to the transitional time before and after menopause. Until recently the medical community didn't recognize this time of gradual change. Women were told they were either "in" or "not in" menopause, leaving no room for being "in-between." Only the strictest laboratory criteria was used to determine this diagnosis. While menopause represents a single point in time when menses stops, it is the result of a gradual process which starts prior to birth and can be felt by physical and emotional changes several years in advance.

By withholding discussion and treatment to only those women "in" menopause, many women in the process of change have faced considerable confusion and needless suffering.

Gradually, perimenopause is being accepted as a true entity. The fact that menopause is only the end point of a transformation that may last from four to six years is finally becoming common knowledge. Although there is a growing body of medical literature related to perimenopause, little of it is in plain language. We, as health care providers, often require women to make important decisions about their health care during this point in their life without providing the necessary background information needed to make those decisions. The available information is oftentimes confusing, which makes a health decision difficult at best.

Use this book as a practical guide. It describes the physical and emotional changes that may take place during perimenopause. It discusses the pros and cons of hormone replacement therapy (HRT), and covers some of the alternative treatments available. This guide also stresses the importance of exercise, proper diet, and stress management. Use this information to be a better prepared, active participant in deciding, along with your health care provider, what course of action is best for you.

Before making a decision on which path to follow, a personal risk assessment should be done. This book will guide you in accomplishing this task and includes the guidelines for filling out this risk assessment.

It is interesting to note that perimenopause is viewed very differently by women around the world. In many traditional cultures, older women hold a position of respect as elders of their community. They remain useful members of their society, respected and looked up to for their wisdom and knowledge. This attitude sharply contrasts with Western cultures, where emphasis is most often placed on youthfulness. Here, the older woman's place of honor has been replaced with a stereotypical picture of an unproductive, non-sensual, hard-to-live-with woman. Western cultures tend to view perimenopause as a negative time in a woman's life, even when the symptoms may be minimal.

Interestingly, several studies show that in cultures where mature women are honored and recognized for their usefulness to society, menopausal symptoms are often minimal or even nonexistent. The better outlook a woman has about herself and her life, the easier time she will have with her passage through perimenopause and eventually through menopause. This is not to say that these physical changes are entirely psychosocial in origin, but it does show how different cultures and your own self-image can alter the intensity of symptoms.

Books are finally beginning to focus on perimenopause in a positive light. They often emphasize that this is an exciting opportunity for you to develop new interests, realize old dreams, and create new ones. It certainly seems time to stop supporting the old myths and make new ones—illuminating the power of this stage of womanhood.

The Ovarian Journey

Menopause has generally been treated by many health care providers as an isolated event rather than the evolving process that it is. This evolving process takes place two to six years prior to the end of both ovulation and monthly periods and is called perimenopause. Because our traditional orientation has been to rely on laboratory results, many women have been told, "You are either in menopause or out of menopause." This type of thinking totally misses the essence of what is taking place in your body.

Menopause actually begins prior to birth. Within the ovary there is a complex system whereby eggs mature—then wither and die. This process occurs on a consistent basis, totally independent of the menstrual cycle. In fact, this process even continues in spite of pregnancy or birth control pill usage.

Prior to your birth, the typical ovary contains five to six million eggs. At birth, the number of eggs has already dropped to one to two million. By the time puberty begins the average egg population is down to around 300,000. During the next thirty-five to forty years of your reproductive life, the numbers will continue to decline at a constant rate. This rate accelerates slightly ten to fifteen years prior to menopause. By the time your periods end—only a few hundred eggs remain.

A quick review of a normal menstrual cycle will be the backdrop upon which I will explain the changes that take place during perimenopause. The typical menstrual cycle is composed of three phases:

▲ Follicular

▲ Ovulatory

▲ Luteal

FOLLICULAR PHASE

Two important events happen during this time. One takes place within the ovary and the other takes place in the uterus. In the ovary, the egg that will eventually be released during ovulation is being selected. This is largely under the influence of a hormone called follicle stimulating hormone or commonly known as FSH.

FSH is a hormone produced by the pituitary gland, which is located within the brain. As the stimulated egg grows, it produces estrogen. As the estrogen level rises, it sends a message back to the brain to stop making FSH since no further stimulation is needed for the egg to grow.

Inside the uterus the newly produced estrogen stimulates a thickening of its lining. This is necessary for implantation of the egg if pregnancy is to occur. Estrogen stimulates the release of another hormone from the pituitary gland called Luteinizing Hormone or LH. LH is responsible for beginning the ovulation process.

OVULATORY PHASE

Responding to estrogen stimulation, the LH rises to a high level commonly called "a spike." The spike sends a signal to the ovary to release the selected egg. Measuring this spike of LH is the primary concept used by ovulation predictor kits that measure infertility. After ovulation the LH causes the ovary to produce the next major hormone, progesterone.

LUTEAL PHASE

Progesterone helps stabilize the thickened lining of the womb. It stimulates the development of a rich blood supply and many nutrient-rich glands, preparing for the possible implantation of an embryo.

After ovulation, progesterone is produced by the cells which surround the released egg. These cells live for nine to eleven days without further stimulation. The hormone that saves them from dying is Human Chorionic Gonadotropin (HCG), which is produced by a developing embryo. HCG continues to stimulate the production of progesterone from the ovary until twelve weeks of gestation. Pregnancy tests measure the HCG level. Without progesterone, the womb lining begins breaking down and your period begins.

FAST FACTS
OVARIES

1. *Life cycle of the ovary (continual decline in available eggs).*
   - ▲ Fetus—*five to six million eggs*
   - ▲ Birth—*one to two million eggs*
   - ▲ Puberty—*300,000 eggs*
   - ▲ Menopause—*A few hundred eggs that are quite resistant to stimulation*

2. *Normal Menstrual Cycle*
   - ▲ *Follicular Phase*
     - • Ovary
       FSH from pituitary stimulates eggs.
       Estrogen increases.
     - • Uterus
       Lining thickens to get ready for implantation.
   - ▲ *Ovulatory*
     - • Ovary
       LH rises rapidly and sparks the release of the dominant egg.
     - • Uterus
       Maximum thickness
   - ▲ *Luteal*
     - • Ovary
       Progesterone is produced by the cells surrounding the site where the egg was released.
     - • Uterus
       Stabilized
   - ▲ *If no pregnancy, the cells producing progesterone begin to wear out.*
     - • *Progesterone levels decrease and menses begins.*
   - ▲ *If pregnancy occurs, the embryo produces HCG.*
     - • *HCG stimulates the eggs to continue to produce progesterone and there is no menses.*

2

Perimenopause

Approximately two to four years before menopause (six to eight years by some authorities), the menstrual cycle begins to lengthen. This occurs because the remaining eggs are of lesser quality and are more resistant to stimulation. Increasing amounts of FSH are needed to coax these eggs to mature and ovulate. Gradually more and more days are needed to raise the FSH to levels high enough to result in ovulation.

Initially FSH and estrogen levels remain in the normal range. Over time, however, the remaining eggs are so resistant that the required FSH levels needed to stimulate the egg become unobtainable, making ovulation either incomplete or impossible. Accompanying this is a decline in both estrogen and progesterone production.

As estrogen and progesterone levels decline, the length of the menstrual cycle becomes variable and is accompanied by irregular bleeding. It must be noted that this process is not always a smooth one. Ovulation may be intermittent. Because of this accompanying symptoms may come and go. Measurement of FSH levels during this time frame may not always correlate with how a woman feels and how her periods are occurring. At this point many health care providers fall short in correctly managing their patients' symptoms. Many feel that if the FSH is not within the menopausal range that their symptoms are psychological, rather than physical. The patient may mistakenly be told, "It's all in your head, you are not going through menopause."

An illustration of what we have just discussed can be seen in the following scenario: It's morning and you are rushing around trying to get ready for work and to also get your family out the door. Suddenly and quite unexpectedly you notice that you are spotting. You can't quite remember when your last period was, but you know you weren't expecting one now. So you put in a tampon or wear a panty liner and keep going. When you check again, the bleeding has stopped, only to return a few days later. Eventually you feel you can't risk having an accident so you start wearing a pad all of the time.

This is the typical way irregular ovulation begins. What you can do to manage it will be discussed in the following chapters, and hopefully these ideas will make your life easier.

FAST FACTS
PERIMENOPAUSE

1. **Your period does not have to stop completely.** *It can become lighter, heavier, shorter, prolonged, or associated with more severe PMS.*

2. **Eggs become more resistant to ovulation.** *Estrogen and progesterone levels decrease.*

   ▲ *Falling progesterone*
   Produces changes in menstrual cycle

   ▲ *Falling estrogen*
   Problems you can see and feel—hot flashes, irritability, insomnia, forgetfulness, vaginal dryness
   Possible unseen problems—osteoporosis, cardiovascular disease

Estrogen Loss

THE SEEN

As estrogen levels begin to decline, numerous changes take place in a woman's body. Some symptoms such as hot flashes, vaginal dryness, and insomnia are readily seen and felt. Other symptoms like osteoporosis and heart disease may develop silently, and are unseen, often until damage has occurred. While both sets of symptoms are the result of the same process, it is helpful to consider these two groups separately. Thinking of the changes in this manner will aid in your decisions concerning treatment options—both traditional and alternative.

HOT FLASHES

Hot flashes are the most well-known symptoms in this group. They most often occur in the evening or at night, although are certainly not limited to these times. With a warm, red flush starting from the chest, the hot flash rises up the neck continuing to the scalp. This is accompanied by perspiration, which may be intense enough to soak your clothes. Finally you may feel a chill as the flush subsides.

The physiological cause for hot flashes is not clearly understood. It is known that estrogen has a regulatory effect on the area of the brain that controls internal body temperature. This area of the brain is called the hypothalamus. Many women even report experiencing a "sense" that a hot flash is about to occur.

Hot flashes occurring at night often cause sleep disturbances, eventually resulting in symptoms of sleep deprivation. This cascade of symptoms precipitated by hot flashes can be thought of as a domino effect. The hot flashes may be severe enough to awaken a woman to find her nightclothes and bedsheets soaked. At other times or for other women, the hot flashes may not be intense enough to awaken her, but simply cause a disturbance in the quality of sleep. Both of these scenarios may lead to chronic sleep deprivation, resulting in moodiness, forgetfulness, and the inability to concentrate. If left untreated, depression may develop. In other words, the single event hot flash results in seemingly unrelated symptoms following behind like dominoes. Oftentimes treating the hot flashes will relieve the other symptoms.

MENTAL EFFECTS

A certain amount of mental slowing is a natural part of aging—for both men and women. Where you once prided yourself on your great memory and ability to think quickly on your feet, now you may need to make lists to remember everything. For some this is accepted as a natural part of life. For others this may be frightening. Anxiety related to mental slowing may be intensified if it is viewed as an early symptom of Alzheimer's disease. The difference between normal and abnormal may be difficult to ascertain. If you are simply a second or two slower in thinking of a word, don't panic, this is normal. If your short-term memory has changed to the extent that you have real difficulty remembering— this may be due to estrogen withdrawal. Some recent studies have suggested a preventive role of estrogen in relation to Alzheimer's, a correlation yet to be fully explored.

VAGINAL EFFECTS

Estrogen also helps to keep the vaginal and vulvar tissues strong, elastic, and moist. With falling estrogen levels many women begin to experience vaginal dryness, irritation, and loss of elasticity in these tissues. This often results in painful intercourse, which may cause you to avoid sex. Similar changes in the tissues surrounding the opening to the bladder (urethra) may result in burning upon urination and also an increased urgency to urinate. This is often misdiagnosed as a chronic yeast or urinary tract infection. Appropriate treatment would be estrogen or a natural alternative, not anti-yeast or antibiotic medications.

Weakening of the vaginal walls may result in less support to the bladder. As the bladder descends, prolapses, or drops into the vagina, there is a change in the angle at which the urethra—the tube that connects the bladder to the outside—inserts into the bladder. The normal angle prevents involuntary urine loss. The changes in supporting tissue cause the angle to be almost straight, which may result in urine loss while exercising, coughing, sneezing, or even laughing. The amount of urine leakage may be mild, requiring only the need for using panty liners, or extreme, possibly preventing a woman from leaving her home.

Kegel Exercises

For many women, the daily use of a panty liner just doesn't work. Some find them uncomfortable to wear. Others may find them too expensive. For others, they aren't really absorbent enough, but they don't want to resort to wearing an "adult diaper" product.

The most common, simple, and least expensive solution to incontinence in women is to learn how to do Kegel exercises, which strengthen the muscular flow of the pelvis, which supports the bladder and womb (or uterus). A few minutes a day performing Kegel exercises may go a long way to helping you with urinary leakage, and may be all that is necessary to solve this embarrassing problem. Doing these exercises can also increase your pleasure during sex. To find the correct muscle that needs to be strengthened, the next time you are urinating, tighten the muscle which stops the urine flow. Once you have felt where that muscle is, that's all there is to doing a Kegel exercise. You can tighten the muscle wherever you are—at the office, driving, while watching TV. Try holding the muscle tight for five seconds, then release. It is important to do the Kegel exercises religiously. For best results they should be done four times a day. To make it easy to remember, anchor the exercises to an activity you perform every day. For instance, you could do one set in the car driving to and from work. Another set could be done at lunch and the last at home in the evening watching TV.

Each set should contain several repetitions. A repetition is one completed exercise. It is helpful to start with five repetitions in each set, then increase to ten, fifteen, and twenty reps as you feel stronger.

EMOTIONAL CHANGES

The combination of mood changes due to sleep deprivation and vaginal irritation due to physical changes in the vulva and vagina many times results in other symptoms including a loss of interest in sexual intimacy. A vicious cycle can be started when the physical discomfort or pain of intercourse intensifies an already depressed mood. This may lead to progressively less interest in sexual activity. Ultimately, a woman may find herself trying to find any excuse to avoid intimacy, thereby avoiding the entire issue. Don't let this happen to you. With less chance of pregnancy, learn to explore the new freedoms opened to you. See the chapter on "Sexual Freedom" for more detailed information.

THE UNSEEN

Osteoporosis and cardiovascular disease are referred to here as unseen because they develop quietly, often going unnoticed. When they finally reveal themselves the damage has generally already been done. Osteoporosis alone accounts for over 40,000 deaths annually, with many more suffering from debility, which is extreme bodily weakness. Cardiovascular disease is the most common cause of death in women over fifty, which comes as a surprise to many women who mistakenly believe it is breast cancer. Fortunately, both osteoporosis and cardiovascular disease can be controlled and many times totally avoided.

OSTEOPOROSIS

With good nutrition and an increased emphasis on exercise and preventive medicine, women's potential lifespans have continued to increase. Unfortunately, accompanying this has been a rise in the incidence of osteoporosis to near epidemic proportions. At present there are some twenty million women affected by osteoporosis. Longevity alone, however, is not the only culprit. Our changing lifestyle also plays an important role. The main offenders are jobs requiring more mental than physical activity, a decrease in dairy product consumption, and an increase in the number of women who smoke.

What is osteoporosis? In order to answer this question, we first need to discuss what is a healthy bone. Structurally, there are two types of bone: a hard thick outer shell, called cortical bone, and a thin delicate internal honeycomb, called trabecular bone. The long bones of the body are primarily made up of cortical bone, whereas the bones of the spine, head of the femur (hip) bone, and the small wrist bones are predominately trabecular. Your bones contain the body's reservoir of calcium. Bones are continually being absorbed and replaced, and for most of our lives a healthy balance exists. After age forty, resorption begins to exceed formation, resulting in bone loss. This process accelerates with the loss of estrogen during peri-menopause. Estrogen normally helps facilitate the transfer of calcium into the bone. Perimenopause, with its associated decline in estrogen levels, makes it more difficult for calcium to enter the bone. Trabecular supportive bone seems to be more sensitive to falling estrogen levels. In fact, during the first twenty years after menopause, there is a 50 percent reduction in the body's total trabecular bone content. This bone loss is accompanied by a 30 percent decrease in cortical bone. The bones of the spine, hips, and wrist are the most affected ones. With the loss of internal support, bones become brittle and break easily. This process has been noted to be greater in Caucasians and Asians but less in the African-American population. Not all of the reduction in bone mass is due to estrogen loss, but it accounts for approximately two-thirds of the bone loss.

What does all of this mean to you? Many times bone loss translates into pain, bone weakness, and also accounts for approximately 40,000 deaths annually. Indeed, 25 percent of women over seventy show some evidence of crush-type fractures in their vertebrae (spinal bones). This leads to a leaning-forward appearance caused by a "hump" deformity of the spine. Accompanying this may be considerable pain. One study showed that the average Caucasian woman could expect to shrink 2 1/2 inches if left untreated. Hip fractures due to osteoporosis begin to occur ten to fifteen years after menopause. Unfortunately, this process frequently is not diagnosed until after a fracture occurs. On a positive note, this process is totally avoidable with planning.

Tests for Osteoporosis

How can you tell if you have decreased bone density and are at risk for osteoporosis? Two tests are currently available to test for osteoporosis. The first is a special X-ray called a DEXA scan (Dual Energy X-ray Absorptionetry). It is available at many hospitals and imaging centers. It takes only a few minutes to perform and uses very low-dose radiation. Standard X-rays do not provide early assessment of fracture risk and are of no use. In fact, 30 percent to 40 percent of the bone density must be lost before a change is seen on standard X-rays. The DEXA scan, on the other hand, can detect much smaller amounts of bone loss. It has been recommended that a woman have a baseline (initial) study between the ages of forty-five and fifty. A follow-up DEXA scan can then be done approximately 1 1/2 years after your last period. Treatment plans may then be tailored to allow for the amount of bone loss present. A significant decrease in bone mass obviously would require a more aggressive treatment plan.

The second test is even newer, more accessible, and less expensive. It consists of a simple urine test that measures the amount of deoxypyridimoline and is called a urine Dpd test. This is a specific marker of bone resorption found in the urine. It costs approximately one quarter of the price of a DEXA scan, making it a very cost effective tool for identifying rapid bone loss. All that is required is to give your health care provider a urine sample that they send off to a lab. As with the DEXA scan, the results of this test can aid in making a decision to initiate the most appropriate treatment plan to stop progressive bone loss. This test can also be used to track your response to your treatment plan. There is also another urine test called the NTx test. Both tests measure molecules released during bone breakdown. (The NTx test measures "Crossed Linked N-telopeptides.")

The DEXA scan does give more information with regard to where the bone resorption is the greatest and helps pinpoint specific locations at risk for fractures. The urine Dpd test is generally considered to be a more overall screening procedure.

The degree of risk a woman has for developing osteoporosis varies, and also depends on specific risk factors. These risk factors include the following:

▲ Family history of osteoporosis

▲ Thinner than average

▲ Smoker

▲ Asian or Caucasian

▲ Consumption of more than two glasses of alcoholic beverages a day

▲ Sedentary lifestyle

▲ Early onset of menopause, generally before age forty-five

From the list of risk factors, it should be noted that quitting smoking and monitoring your alcohol consumption are two good places to start in order to prevent osteoporosis. Also consider adding calcium supplements to your daily diet. The average diet supplies approximately 500 mg of calcium daily. Women taking hormone replacement therapy should add 500 mg of calcium per day to bring their daily total to 1000 mg. These amounts have been shown to be necessary to reduce bone loss. Menopausal women not on estrogen replacement should add 1000 mg of calcium per day (bringing the total to 1500 mg) due to the less efficient absorption by your bones.

Many commercial calcium supplements are available and can be found in several different forms. Calcium carbonate seems to be the most easily absorbed form of calcium on the market today. Don't be surprised if you experience some increased intestinal gas and slight abdominal bloating when you use calcium carbonate. Another excellent source of additional calcium can be found in chewable antacid tablets. You may find these less expensive, too.

Weight-bearing exercise—which includes walking, aerobics, running, or lifting weights—is one of the best preventative measures you can take to head off osteoporosis. No special or expensive equipment is necessary, except for a pair of well-fitting, supportive shoes. If your finances and space constraints allow it, you may wish to consider purchasing a treadmill. There are some models that fold up for easier storage.

While swimming or water aerobics aren't technically weight-bearing exercises, they are often a wise choice for women who may be overweight or have joint pain or inflammation, including those suffering from arthritis.

However, if evidence of osteoporosis is shown through diagnostic testing, consideration should be given to starting either hormone replacement therapy (see the following chapter for more information) or taking alendronate. Alendronate is a nonhormonal medication approved for the treatment of osteoporosis. It works by reducing the activity of the cells that cause bone loss (osteoclast). This allows bone formation to exceed resorption, leading to progressive gains in bone mass. In order to ensure optimum absorption into the bloodstream, alendronate must be taken orally in a prescribed manner. It is taken once a day—every day—first thing in the morning with plain water only. Mineral water, coffee, tea, or juice decrease absorption and should not be taken with medication. Alendronate is only effective when taken on an empty stomach, preferably thirty minutes before your first meal, beverage, or before taking any other medication. Waiting longer than thirty minutes will improve the absorption rate even more. It is also advisable that you do not lie down for at least thirty minutes after taking alendronate. This will help to avoid irritation of the esophagus and prevent heartburn. If you happen to miss a dose, you should not take it later in the day. Simply resume your normal schedule the next morning.

It is extremely important to remember that alendronate will treat your osteoporosis only as long as you continue taking it. Side effects from taking alendronate are usually mild and rarely prevent women from continuing treatment. The side effects include:

▲ Some stomach discomfort

▲ Heartburn

▲ Nausea

▲ Bloated feeling

▲ Constipation or diarrhea

▲ Gas

Remember, alendronate only treats osteoporosis and is not considered to be a substitute for hormone replacement therapy, which also offers protection against heart disease. Please read the following chapter for much more discussion on hormone replacement therapy.

CARDIOVASCULAR DISEASE

Ask women what disease they fear the most after the age of fifty, and often their response will be "breast cancer." The truth is, heart disease, not breast cancer is the most common cause of death after age fifty for women. This misconception is likely due to the medical community's emphasis on men and heart disease. There is no denying that men in general are at high risk for heart disease. The difference between men and women's risk is not in degree but in the time of onset. During the reproductive years, estrogen helps to protect women from coronary artery disease. Their risk lags behind men as much as ten to fifteen years. This lag mistakenly gave physicians the impression that women were at lower risk during their whole life. Research was then directed almost exclusively toward prevention and treatment for men. Unfortunately, this has led to delays in diagnosing heart disease in many women. It also gave women a false sense of security, causing them to become complacent about monitoring for warning signs and starting a healthy heart program.

Estrogen's protection relates to its beneficial effect on fat metabolism or more specifically its effect on cholesterol. Estrogen is responsible for increasing the amount of HDL-cholesterol (good cholesterol) while decreasing LDL-cholesterol (bad cholesterol which can lead to coronary artery disease). HDL (high-density lipoprotein) cholesterol is responsible for carrying fat away from the blood vessels. LDL (low-density lipoprotein) cholesterol causes the blood vessels to become blocked with fat deposits called plaque. The accumulation of this plaque is called atherosclerosis. The best test of cholesterol levels is a fasting lipid profile.

Recent studies have also shown estrogen to have a direct effect on the walls of the coronary arteries, preventing them from spasm and constriction. This is important because it maintains the normal blood flow to the heart muscle with less chance of obstruction.

Normally during your late forties, LDL levels begin to rise. At perimenopause these levels increase rapidly. With this rise in LDL, the risk of heart disease doubles. Accompanying decreased levels of estrogen, there are other risk factors that may accelerate the risk of developing heart disease. Some of these risk factors are:

- ▲ Hypertension
- ▲ Smoking
- ▲ Diabetes
- ▲ Family history of heart disease including—
  - • Premature heart disease before age sixty in your mother or sister
  - • Premature heart disease before age fifty in your father or brother
- ▲ Obesity (20 percent or more over your ideal weight)
- ▲ Increased stress
- ▲ Lack of regular exercise
- ▲ Elevated total cholesterol with a non-favorable ratio of HDL to LDL or elevated triglycerides
- ▲ Race
  - • Highest incidence in African-American women
  - • Next highest incidence in Caucasian women

Refer to the chapters on exercise and eating to stay fit for ways to decrease your risk of heart disease.

BY WAY OF REFERENCES:

I. Blood Pressure (mm/Hg)

	SYSTOLIC (top number)	DIASTOLIC (bottom number)
Normal	less than 130	less than 85
High Normal	130–139	85–89
Hypertension	140–159	90–99

II. Cholesterol/Lipoprotein Profile

Normal

Total Cholesterol	Less than 200 mg/dL
HDL-Cholesterol	Greater than 50 mg/dL
LDL-Cholesterol	Less than 130 mg/dL
Triglycerides	Less than 250 mg/dL

FAST FACTS

ESTROGEN LOSS

1. *Domino theory*
   - ▲ *Hot flashes at night* → *restless sleep* → *chronic sleep deprivation* → *memory loss / fatigue / depression / feeling of worthlessness*

2. *Vaginal dryness*
   - ▲ *Chronic irritation and painful intercourse, urinary frequency and burning*

3. *Less pelvic support*
   - ▲ *Urine loss*
   - ▲ *Kegels*

4. *Emotional changes*
   - ▲ *Sleep deprivation and physical changes* → *depression*

5. *Osteoporosis*
   - ▲ *After age forty, breakdown of bone exceeds formation.*
   - ▲ *Bone breakdown accelerates with the loss of estrogen.*
   - ▲ *Estrogen normally facilitates the transfer of calcium into the bones.*
   - ▲ *There are two types of bone: hard outer cortical, and inner delicate supportive trabecular.*
   - ▲ *During the first twenty years after menopause there is a 50 percent reduction in trabecular and a thirty percent decrease in cortical, leading to pain and debility from deformity and fracture.*

▲ *Screening Tests*
  • *DEXA Scan*
  • *Urine Dpd test*
▲ *Prevention*
  • *Weight-bearing exercise*
  • *Stop smoking*
  • *Increase dietary calcium*
    Add 1000 mg per day without estrogen replacement
    Add 500 mg per day taking estrogen replacement
▲ *Treatment*
  • *Estrogen replacement*
  • *Alendronate*

6. Cardiovascular Disease

▲ *Reproductive years: women lag ten years behind men in rate of coronary artery disease and twenty years behind in rate of heart attack and sudden death.*

▲ *Menopause: decreased estrogen results in a rise in LDL-cholesterol levels, with a doubling of heart disease risk.*

▲ *Prevention*
  • *Decrease dietary fat intake to no more than 30 percent daily calories.*
  • *Twenty minutes of dedicated aerobic-type exercise, three times a week (walking, bike riding, stair stepper, etc.).*
  • *Quit Smoking!*
  • *Consider estrogen replacement—especially with a strong family history of heart disease and low family history of breast cancer.*

Hormone Replacement Therapy (HRT)

Replacing your lost estrogen may help relieve hot flashes, insomnia, and vaginal dryness. HRT may also help to prevent heart disease and osteoporosis. While its use is widely supported in the medical community, it is not for everyone and not without risk. The decision to use hormone replacement therapy is personal and complex.

Some common questions I am often asked by women considering estrogen replacement are:

▲ Will I continue to have a period?

▲ How long will I need to continue HRT?

▲ What happens if I stop taking HRT?

▲ Does HRT increase my risk for cancer?

This chapter will answer these questions and discuss both the benefits and drawbacks of HRT. Also presented is an explanation of the types of hormones most commonly used and how they are administered. With this information you will be better prepared to take an active role in deciding, along with your health care provider, what is best for you. Again, let me state that hormone replacement therapy is not for everyone either by choice or because of potential risks. You may also wish to consider alternative methods of treatment that are presented in later chapters.

There are a number of women who have the mistaken notion that if they start estrogen replacement therapy they must continue it indefinitely or suffer some ill effects. While it may be advantageous to continue HRT long term, there is absolutely no reason to believe that once started you must continue it forever. In fact, some studies show that the greatest benefit in preventing osteoporosis is when estrogen is taken for the first five to ten years after menopause. While some benefit continues after this, the benefit is not as great. Additionally, one of the largest studies concerning the potential risk of breast cancer associated with estrogen showed no increase for up to five years when taken at the lowest effective dose. With this in mind, a woman could elect to start estrogen knowing she is safe (according to the literature) up to five years and at that point reevaluate the most current literature.

You may feel that your symptoms aren't bad enough to justify taking hormone therapy. Although the symptoms of estrogen withdrawal can range from mild discomfort to significant inter- ference with your daily routines, the increased risks for cardiovas- cular disease and osteoporosis remain the most important things to be taken into consideration.

Unwanted side effects of estrogen replacement include:

▲ Breast tenderness

▲ Headaches

▲ Stomach upset

▲ Fluid retention

▲ Leg cramps

Because of these side effects, many women either stop taking hormone therapy after a short trial period or never begin taking it. What needs to be understood is that there is no single dosing sched- ule or type of hormone for everyone, but a therapy should be cus- tomized for you. It is not uncommon to make three to four phone calls or visits to your health care provider before the right combina- tion of dose and schedule are found. It is certainly in everyone's interest for a woman to be encouraged to call if she has a problem or question. The primary reason so many of the women who initiate hormone replacement therapy stop soon after is because they were afraid to question their health care provider. This shouldn't be and if you don't feel comfortable with discussing any subject with your health care provider, don't just simply stop treatment or stop going to appointments, but consider finding a health care provider with whom you feel comfortable.

The primary goal of effective hormone replacement therapy is to find the lowest dose of hormones with the least amount of side effects, but that is still able to control your symptoms while helping to prevent heart disease and osteoporosis. Fortunately, today we have greater flexibility in finding not only the best dose and schedule for taking estrogen and progestin, but in also selecting the best type suited to you.

There are many estrogens on the market today. None, however, appear to be clearly superior in benefits when compared to others. Some are derived from natural sources, such as from animals or plants, and others are synthetic. Each has its own subtle differences in how the body handles the hormone. The variety in these available estrogens does allow for greater flexibility in finding the one that is right for you.

There is a growing body of support for using a natural estrogen combination pill in place of the commercially available estrogen pills naturally derived or synthetic. This combination estrogen pill is both safe and effective for estrogen replacement. Since this is rather new some discussion is in order.

The theory behind a combination estrogen pill is based on the knowledge that what we call "estrogen" in a woman's body is really made up of three distinct estrogens. Chemically they differ only slightly but they differ dramatically in their impact on a woman's body. The three estrogens are: estriol, which makes up 60 to 80 percent of the total estrogens and is the least powerful; estrone, which consists of 10 to 20 percent of the total and is moderately potent; and estradiol, which makes up the remaining 10 to 20 percent of the total and is the most powerful.

For many years, estriol was ignored by researchers since it was believed to be the weakest and least significant estrogen. Actually, estriol was found to be the most important because of its less potent effect. By virtue of its "weaker" effect it exerts a moderating effect on the other two estrogens and is felt to be important in protecting the body against estrogen-associated cancers.

Traditional estrogen replacement, even from "natural" origins (animal/plant), does not deliver estriol. Estrogen derived from horses, although natural, is 75 to 80 percent estrone. Several of the "natural" estrogens commercially available from plants are almost 100 percent estradiol.

Triple estrogen or "triest" is not available in every drugstore like its more commercial counterparts. You must take the prescription from your health care provider to a pharmacist who is still interested in the art of compounding (preparing or mixing) pharmaceuticals. The component parts of this mixture come under the same close scrutiny of the USP (United States Pharmacopeia Standards of Purity) as any other medicine. The compounding pharmacist mixes estriol, estrone, and estradiol into a single gel cap or pill reproducing the same ratio each has in a woman's body. The usual dose of triest is 2.5 mg/day. This can be taken in a cyclic fashion with micronized oral progesterone or on a continuous regimen.

In 1979 a Northern California physician, John R. Lee, MD, started researching and prescribing natural progesterone. Like natural estrogen it is derived from wild yam (dioscorea). In his literature he points out that natural as opposed to synthetic progesterone not only has fewer side effects (e.g., fluid retention, bloating, swelling, breast tenderness, weight gain), but was found to be more important than estrogen in combating osteoporosis. His research suggests that where estrogen prevents further bone loss, natural progesterone may actually lead to new bone formation.

Natural micronized progesterone is also only available from a compounding pharmacist. The usual dosage is 100 mg on days 16 to 25 of the cycle, or 50 mg daily.

To locate a compounding pharmacist you may contact:

International Academy of Compounding Pharmacists
P.O. Box 1365
Sugar Land, Texas 77487
Telephone: 800-927-4227
Fax: 713-495-0602
Internet: www.iacp.com/iacp

There are some new estrogens that will be available soon. They fall into a new category called "designer estrogens." Many feel that they will allow more women to feel comfortable about choosing HRT. The idea behind this new generation of estrogens is that they take on the good qualities of estrogen, while not causing the bad side effects. I would caution you, however, to be just as thorough in your investigation of these estrogens. They are so new that there hasn't been time to do any studies yet on possible long-term side effects or risks. There is also some suggestion that they may make your body resistant to cancer-fighting drugs, since some designer estrogens are similar to these drugs in composition.

Progestins are also available from both synthetic and natural sources which allows for greater customizing of your hormone therapy to best fill your needs. The manner in which estrogens and progestins are taken together can also be tailored to your needs. You can take separate estrogen and progestin pills; estrogen patches with oral progestin; or one of the new combination pills, which contain both estrogen and progestin. Again, it's not a question of what's best for the general population, but for you as an individual. This requires some open dialogue between you and your health care provider.

Whether a woman chooses to use estrogen pills instead of patches is largely a matter of personal preference. In some circumstances, the patch may offer some advantages. This is especially true for women with liver disease or certain blood clotting disorders. The estrogen in the patch, unlike that in tablets, does not require passage through nor metabolism by the liver. Women who suffer from intestinal upset when taking estrogen and women who have had a prior hysterectomy may also find the patches to be a pleasant alternative. Following a hysterectomy, a woman does not need to take progestin to balance estrogen and a patch may be all she needs.

Some of the older patches were bulkier and required twice-per-week replacement. They didn't stay attached very well during exercise or while in saunas, hot tubs, or swimming pools. The newer patches are very sheer, replaced only once a week, and were specifically designed to stay attached in steam, heat, and during exercise.

It should also be noted that estrogen patches, like estrogen pills, come in several different dose forms that can be individualized to a woman's needs. Unlike some new combination estrogen/progestin pills, there are presently no combination patches. Therefore, unless you have had a hysterectomy and don't require progestin, you will still need to take progestins orally. This can be done either cyclically or continuously. However, you may be able to use alternative therapies in place of progestin. Please see pages 43-44 for more information.

Many women question if they will get their period again every month. Answering this question is one of the greatest challenges while discussing hormone replacements. The ovaries of women who have recently stopped having periods may continue to produce a small amount of estrogen. When you add an estrogen supplement to this "endogenous estrogen," the total estrogen level may be high enough to cause irregular bleeding. In order to avoid this it is sometimes less stressful and more convenient to do estrogen and progesterone in a cyclic fashion and have a regular period. As this cyclic bleeding becomes less and less heavy you may consider taking continuous estrogen and progesterone with no further bleeding.

Estrogens and progestins can be used in either a cyclic or continuous fashion. Each method has its own advantages. The cyclic method involves taking estrogen for twenty-five days a month or continuously. The progestin is then added for ten to fourteen days either at the beginning of the cycle or during the second half of the cycle. This can involve either using separate estrogen and progestin tablets, patches, progestin pills/capsules, or a single pill combining both. Starting on the first day of the month may help you to stay on a regular schedule. Regardless of how you combine the estrogen and progestin though, if taken in a cyclic fashion, you will have a cyclic, predictable, withdrawal bleeding. For a younger woman who may be experiencing irregular periods or just recently stopped having periods, this may be the preferred choice. The reasoning is that if you attempt continuous therapy at this stage, unpredictable breakthrough bleeding may occur. With a busy lifestyle, a predictable pattern is usually more acceptable and easier to plan for.

The continuous method involves a daily intake of both estrogen and progestin. Taken in this manner, the daily progestin dose is lower than that taken during cyclic hormone replacement therapy. This has the advantage of lessening the potential progestin side effects of water retention, bloating, and premenstrual-like feelings. The other benefit is that after an initial adjustment period of four to six months, you no longer have any withdrawal bleeding. Again, although this is an appealing benefit, it may not work as well for a woman still having regular periods, irregular bleeding, or who has just finished having periods.

One reason for taking progestin along with estrogen is for its protective effect on the lining of the womb (uterus). The body manufactures both progestin and estrogen during your reproductive years and, with hormone replacement therapy, we are simply restoring that natural balance. While the potential for estrogen, when taken alone, to cause uterine cancer has been well documented, adding progestin helps to prevent this cancer from occurring. The role of progestin having a similar protective effect against breast cancer has not been definitively shown. There has been only one study which suggested a possible beneficial effect, and this result was not seen in subsequent studies. Currently, most reproductive endocrinologists feel that estrogen can be taken alone only in a woman who has had a hysterectomy.

To avoid possible stomach upset, it is helpful to take estrogen and progestin later in the day with a good-sized meal. Some authorities have also suggested some alternative methods of estrogen delivery to avoid stomach upset. Estrogen and progestin pills, capsules, and suppositories may be inserted vaginally, enabling them to be absorbed through the vaginal wall. This is helpful for women who can't tolerate the hormones orally or who may be allergic to the adhesive used on patches. The drawback of this method is the potential for incomplete absorption resulting in lower blood levels of the hormones.

For women who either choose not to take hormones or must decline for medical reasons, vaginal estrogen cream is available. Vaginal estrogen cream may be administered with a ring which time releases the estrogen, allowing it to work locally in the vagina. Both the vaginal cream and estrogen ring work quickly in the vaginal area to reverse the drying effect of estrogen withdrawal. With estrogen withdrawal, the lining of the vagina becomes thin, dry, and less flexible. When using vaginal estrogen, the vaginal wall regains its normal thickness, becomes more flexible, and lubricated. This in turn leads to greater support for the bladder and urethra, helping to control urinary stress incontinence. Less drying irritation helps to relieve and prevent burning on urination, increased urinary frequency, urinary urgency, and painful intercourse. Vaginal estrogen may also be added to hormone replacement therapy when an additional localized amount is needed. This avoids an increase in the amount of estrogen taken orally or through a patch.

Women who have been without estrogen for some time, and who have already developed symptoms of vaginal dryness and irritation, may experience some breast tenderness when beginning to use estrogen cream. Since the vaginal wall has already become thin, some estrogen is initially absorbed into the bloodstream. This amount will decrease as the wall regains its normal thickness. Localized burning and discomfort may be experienced until the estrogen has had time to heal the tissues. This irritation from the cream should not be misinterpreted as an allergy to the estrogen. Before discontinuing therapy, it is advisable to discuss your symptoms with your health care provider. It is important to remember that vaginal estrogen cream only works locally and does not offer any protection against osteoporosis or heart disease.

Many women wonder if taking estrogen increases their risk for breast cancer. Certainly the risk of breast cancer weighs heavily on the minds of all women—and with good reason. It is the number one cancer found in American women, second only to lung cancer as a cause of cancer deaths in American women. Unfortunately, the number of new cases of breast cancer appears to be on an increase every year.

There is good news as well. With the better detection and treatment options that are available today, the survival rates have greatly improved. Presently, the five-year survival rate for a woman whose breast cancer was found before it spread to other areas is greater than 90 percent.

Keeping all of this in mind, it is not difficult to understand that anything that even remotely could be thought to increase a woman's risk for developing breast cancer is avoided. For this reason, many women decline hormone replacement therapy, and of those who do start, many choose to stop shortly thereafter.

At present it is not known for sure whether or not long-term use of estrogen increases a woman's risk of breast cancer. However, it is known that short-term use, considered to be five years or less, doesn't appear to increase your risk.

Three large studies regarding hormone replacement therapy have received the most attention. These studies are: The Nurses

Health Study (120,000 women), The Western Washington State Study, and the American Cancer Society Study (600,000 women).

The Nurses Health Study began in 1976, and questionnaires were sent every two years to track any change in hormone exposure of the study participants. They found a small but positive increase in relative risk between long-term (longer than five years) estrogen use and breast cancer. No association was found with the short-term use of estrogen (five years or less).

The Western Washington State Study started in the late 1980s and interviewed women who had developed breast cancer. Their findings were directly opposite from those in the Nurses Health Study. Here, no relationship was found between estrogen use and breast cancer. Also no difference in risk was found in using estrogen alone or in combination with progestin.

The most recent of these studies is the American Cancer Society's study. This study specifically asked women about estrogen use for non-contraceptive purposes. They actually found a 16 percent reduction in breast cancer and improved survivorship of those who had breast cancer among the estrogen users.

As one can see, these studies show conflicting results. No one at this time can give a definite "yes" or "no" answer as to whether the risk of breast cancer is actually increased by estrogen use. We do know the following information:

▲ In the studies that show an increased relative risk of breast cancer, the magnitude is small (1.3 percent increase relative risk).

▲ Although we know that there is a high risk between taking unopposed estrogen (estrogen alone without progesterone) and developing endometrial (uterine) cancer, this same level of risk does not appear to exist in causing breast cancer.

▲ Any risk should be balanced against potential benefits, especially in a woman with a strong family history of osteoporosis or heart disease.

▲ Data is consistent in showing little if any increase in risk with short-term estrogen use (five years or less).

The real issue is whether there is a modest increase in breast cancer among long-term users, and this answer remains unclear at this time. However, with the improved study design and data collection we have today, we know that the information that will be available in five to eight years will greatly overshadow the current information. Then women will have more straightforward information for making decisions.

To conclude, a woman at low individual risk should feel comfortable in taking estrogen short term for up to five years. With this choice she should commit to reevaluating her decision on a yearly basis with her health care provider, after examining any new data.

Breast cancer screening can't be overlooked regardless of your decision about taking estrogen. When done individually, mammograms and breast self-exams may miss small tumors but when used in combination they provide a sensitive screening mechanism with over 80 percent accuracy.

Unfortunately, good intentions fall by the wayside after awhile and self-exams are often forgotten and mammograms postponed. I've found it helpful to suggest that you "anchor" your breast self-exams to a specific, recurrent monthly event. Women still having a regular period may choose to use this as a cue to remember to perform the self-exam at the end of her period. It isn't advisable to do a breast self-exam during your period, as many women develop lumps that disappear after bleeding stops. Women no longer having periods can use either the first day of the month or the date of their birthday to remember.

The American Cancer Society recommends that a screening mammogram be performed by age thirty-five, or age thirty for women with a first-degree relative—mother, sister, daughter—with breast cancer. Starting at age forty, mammograms should be performed every other year until age fifty, then yearly after that. Periodically there are articles either refuting the necessity of mammograms, or pointing to the X-ray risk. However, none of these has been significant enough to change the recommendations of the American Cancer Society. The amount of X-ray exposure from the machines available today is minimal.

FAST FACTS

HORMONE REPLACEMENT THERAPY

1. *Estrogen replacement*
   - ▲ Controls hot flashes which can lead to sleep disturbances, mood swings, and forgetfulness
   - ▲ Prevents osteoporosis and decreases the risk of heart disease

2. *Estrogen*
   - ▲ Tablets, patches, and vaginal cream
   - ▲ Different doses and sources available

3. *Progestins*
   - ▲ Women with uteruses must balance the estrogen with a progestin
   - ▲ Available in tablets, gel caps, and vaginal suppositories
   - ▲ Different doses and sources available

4. *Hormone replacement options*
   - ▲ Cyclic
     - • Useful for women still having periods or recently stopped
     - • Regular bleeding with this method
   - ▲ Continuous
     - • Has no withdrawal bleeding
     - • Works better for women who are definitely menopausal (have been without a period for at least a year)
     - • Women who have had a hysterectomy may take estrogen alone daily.

5. Cancer risk studies

▲ Endometrial (uterine) Cancer

- Studies have shown that when estrogen is taken by itself, it has been associated with an increased risk of cancer of the uterus.
- Adding progestin for at least ten days during the cycle prevents this from occurring.
- Two exceptions are:
  1. A woman having regular periods who develops flashes. Her withdrawal bleeding every month reflects sufficient progesterone production in her body. She can add estrogen alone.
  2. After hysterectomy

▲ Breast Cancer

- Current literature is less clear to what degree estrogen use increases risk of breast cancer.
- What the studies have shown is that risk does not appear to be increased when estrogen is taken for five years or less.
- The information we will have available in the next five years will greatly overshadow what we know presently.
- It is certainly reasonable to start estrogen replacement and review the literature yearly with your health care provider.

CHAPTER

5

Alternative Therapies

Is estrogen replacement therapy really necessary? Estrogen is certainly not for all women. The reason may be individual choice or preference, or because of a pre-existing medical condition which precludes using estrogen. The answer is a personal one and one you must feel comfortable with. We have discussed the pros and cons of current medical treatment. Following is a discussion of some "traditional alternatives." My hope is that this information will aid you in your own personal decision.

In cultures where perimenopause is considered to be a natural, positive part of life rather than a negative event, hot flashes and other symptoms are frequently milder, sometimes even nonexistent. Historically, the West has treated menopause more as a deficiency disease than as a natural physiologic process. Referring to hot flashes, mood swings, and vaginal dryness as "symptoms" rather than signs of estrogen withdrawal has supported the concept of a "disease process." The observation that the intensity of hot flashes varies with sociocultural attitude toward menopause raises questions concerning the necessity of taking estrogen. Might not a change in attitude, along with good nutritional support, exercise, and an assessment of your potential cardiovascular and osteoporosis risks be a more logical first step?

One of the most detailed studies of cultural effects on menopause involved rural Mayan Indians. Fifty-two postmenopausal women underwent physical exams, blood hormone level testing, and bone density studies. Not one woman reported hot flashes or other menopausal signs. No evidence of osteoporosis was found in spite of similar hormone levels when compared to women living in the United States. Mayan women have a positive view of menopause as they now are seen as respected elders in their community while being free from childbearing responsibilities.

Certainly this is a small study and there are many variables that must be taken into consideration. But it does serve to illustrate that the way a woman's culture perceives menopause may have a significant impact on how she as an individual feels physically.

We have already seen how hot flashes are not only uncomfortable but by disturbing sleep, may lead to a myriad of other problems. Because of this, a good deal of the alternative medicine literature concerns itself with relieving this problem. Hot flashes are usually the worst during the first two years of estrogen withdrawal. However, there does seem to be a great deal of variation. Some women experience hot flashes for several years. While altered function within the hypothalamus appears to be the most likely cause, the exact mechanism is not known. The hypothalamus is located in the central part of the brain where it is surrounded by the limbic system, which controls emotion. The limbic system is a term applied to a group of main structures associated with emotion and behavior. Specifically it seems to recognize upsets in a person's physical and psychological condition that might threaten survival. The hypothalamus is also connected to the pituitary gland. The pituitary gland produces regulatory hormones which control the function of the thyroid, ovaries, and adrenal glands. The hypothalamus in this way forms a bridge between the nervous, emotional, and hormonal systems. It is responsible for controlling body temperature, metabolic rate, sleep patterns, reaction to stress, libido, and release of pituitary regulatory hormones.

Endorphins are substances critical to the proper functioning of the hypothalamus. They are sometimes referred to as the body's natural painkillers and tranquilizers and have an overall calming effect. Exercise and acupuncture are both thought to increase and promote endorphin production and therefore may indirectly relieve symptoms of perimenopause, such as hot flashes.

EXERCISE

Researchers in Sweden investigated the possibility of impaired endorphin activity as a major factor in producing hot flashes. This study was designed to investigate if increasing endorphin output through regular exercise would decrease the intensity and frequency of hot flashes. They compared seventy-nine post-menopausal women who exercised regularly to a group of non-exercising women, which was the control group. Both groups completed questionnaires, which included questions about the frequency of hot flashes and asked them to rate them as mild, moderate, or severe. The women who exercised were also asked about the frequency and intensity of physical activity. The results showed that dedicated physical exercise had a positive influence on decreasing the frequency and severity of hot flashes. The most exciting news was that the women in the exercise group who reported the absence of hot flashes exercised only a minimum of 3 1/2 hours per week. This appears to be the critical level, since women who exercised for shorter periods than that did experience some hot flashes. The intensity of hot flashes, however, was lower than those experienced by the non-exercising control group. Since endorphin levels were not directly measured, it cannot definitively be stated that endorphins caused this response. However, a strong implication may be made. Regular exercise is not only vital in preventing osteoporosis and promoting a healthy heart, but may aid in controlling or possibly eliminating hot flashes. Other health benefits of regular exercise during perimenopause include:

▲ A reduction in blood pressure

▲ Decreased blood cholesterol levels

▲ Increased energy

▲ Improved ability to deal with stress

▲ An improved body image with greater self-esteem

See the "Exercise the Mind and Body" chapter for more information.

DIET

Some dietary changes are useful in controlling the effects of estrogen withdrawal. Dietary therapy for controlling hot flashes and vaginal dryness has centered primarily around a group of foods rich in substances called phytoestrogens. Phytoestrogens are estrogens derived from plants, literally plant estrogens. When ingested, they appear to function much like human estrogens, although phytoestrogens are only 1 to 2 percent as potent. These include soy, fennel, celery, parsley, nuts, seeds, and high-lignin flaxseed oil. Of these foods, soy has gotten the most attention. A mild estrogenic effect is produced by the isoflavones and phytosterols found in soybeans. One cup of soybeans provides 300 mg of isoflavone, which is approximately equivalent to 0.45 mg of conjugated estrogen. "Conjugated" refers to conjugated equine estrogen, which is the most commercially available form of estrogen (brand name is Premarin®). It is derived from horse urine. A higher intake of phytoestrogens is thought to explain why hot flashes and other perimenopausal signs are rarely seen in cultures with a plant-based diet high in soy products.

Fennel is particularly high in phytoestrogens. To make a tea out of fennel, pour a cup of boiling water over one to two teaspoons of crushed seeds, then steep for ten minutes. You may drink this tea two to three times a day. Whole fennel seeds can be found in the spice section of almost any grocery store.

Plant lignins are compounds found not only to relieve hot flashes (due to their mild estrogenic effect) but also believed by many naturopaths to have a protective effect against breast cancer. The theory is that plant lignins have a weaker estrogenic effect than the body's estrogen. By competing for and taking up (binding to) the estrogen receptors in the breast tissue, plant lignins are actually exerting an overall decrease of estrogen activity in the breast. High-lignan flaxseed oil contains 100 times the amount of lignan found in other plant sources. One tablespoon per day is the usual recommended dose.

SUPPLEMENTS

Vitamin E in doses of 800 IU taken daily has been found to decrease the intensity and frequency of hot flashes. Once the hot flashes have subsided, the dose is then reduced to 400 IU a day. Although there is no scientific evidence to support this, there are many testimonials to its effectiveness. Women with diabetes, high blood pressure, rheumatic heart disease, or those taking digitalis should consult with their health care provider before increasing dietary Vitamin E. Also you should not exceed 1000 IU a day without consulting a qualified nutritionist. Discontinue use immediately if you notice blurred vision or any other symptoms. Nutritionists recommend that for best absorption Vitamin E should be taken with a B-complex vitamin, 500 mg of Vitamin C, 25 mcg of selenium (a trace mineral), and some food containing unsaturated fat. A discussion of types of fats is found in the "Eating to Stay Fit" chapter.

Calcium is extremely important to maintain strong, healthy bones and to prevent osteoporosis. Good food sources of calcium are yogurt and other milk products, almonds, sesame seeds and sesame products, and most dark green leafy vegetables. Spinach, chard, and turnip greens are all excellent sources of calcium. Herbs that provide high amounts of calcium include oats, nettle, dandelion greens, mustard seed, horsetail, chickweed, and water cress. There are some excellent natural calcium/mineral supplements made from herbs and organic sources. Biochelated mineral supplements are more expensive but are thought to be absorbed better by the body. You may also wish to supplement your diet with calcium pills or calcium carbonate antacid tablets. See the previous chapter for a more in-depth discussion of calcium.

HEALTHFUL HERBS

For centuries women have used herbs containing phytoestrogens for the relief of PMS, menstrual cramps (dysmenorrhea), menstrual irregularities, and menopausal symptoms. While controlled prospective studies have yet to be performed, it is difficult to ignore the favorable results over the past several hundred years. One advantage phytoestrogens appear to have over synthetic and natural estrogens is an apparent lack of promoting cancer. Unopposed estrogen (without progesterone) has been associated with causing endometrial (uterine) cancer. And there is a suggestion that estrogen may be associated with an increased risk of breast cancer. But no such association has been reported with phytoestrogens. The risk of clot formation (thrombo-embolic disease) and gallbladder disease also appears to be absent.

It is interesting to note that the same herbs (such as dong quai) are recommended for conditions of excess estrogen (PMS) as well as times of low estrogen (perimenopause). The explanation offered is that phytoestrogens exert an estrogen effect that is quite weak. It is only 2 percent as strong as natural-occurring estrogen. This weak estrogen effect allows it to perform a balancing function. In situations of low estrogen it is strong enough to make up for the deficit. In high estrogen states the phytoestrogens compete for and bind to receptors, weakening the estrogen. The overall effect dilutes and lowers estrogen in the body.

The herbs found most useful for controlling hot flashes and vaginal dryness are dong quai (*Angelica sinensis*), black cohosh (*Cimicifuga racemosa*), licorice root (*Glycyrrhiza gubra*), and chasteberry (*Vitex agnus-castus*). While useful individually, you may find that combining several of them increases their effectiveness.

DONG QUAI (*ANGELICA SINENSIS*)

In Asia, Dong Quai is regarded as the primary female herbal remedy. It is useful for both hot flashes and menstrual cramps. Its beneficial effect on hot flashes is believed to be due to a combination of both a mild estrogenic effect and its ability to stabilize blood vessels. Dong quai is available in several forms: tinctures (extracts), powder, tablets, whole root, and whole-pressed root. The usual dose is two tablets twice a day, or 1/4 teaspoon of extract mixed in tea or hot water and drunk twice a day.

BLACK COHOSH (*CIMICIFUGA RACEMOSA*)

Black cohosh is widely used by Native Americans, particularly the Algonquins and Colonists, and grows wild from Maine to Michigan. By the 1800s, its beneficial qualities were so widely known that it became a popular commercial product for women. Most notable was the fact that it was the main ingredient in Lydia Pinkham's famous "vegetable compound and tea" used to treat women's "spells."

Popular in Europe for over forty years, the Germans have refined and standardized the black cohosh compound. Since 1956, over 1 1/2 million menopausal German women have successfully taken it without side effects. Clinical studies there have shown it to be useful in relieving both hot flashes and vaginal dryness.

Black cohosh is standardized to contain 1 mg of 27-deoxy-actein (the active substance) per tablet. The usual dose is one to two tablets twice daily (2–4 mg/day). Studies have shown this to produce symptomatic relief comparable to HRT, and apparently without the risk. To make a tea you would place one teaspoon of dried root in a cup of water and boil. Simmer for 10 minutes and drink the tea up to three times a day. Two to four ml of extract can also be taken three times a day. Do not take black cohosh if you have an irregular heartbeat since it may aggravate your condition.

CHASTEBERRY (*VITEX AGNUS-CASTUS*)

British women have found this herb to be quite useful in controlling hot flashes. It is believed to work by balancing both estrogen and progesterone levels. A tea is made by pouring one cup of boiling water over one teaspoon of fresh berries. Steep for ten minutes. You may drink up to three cups of the tea a day. One ml of extract can also be taken three times a day. Note that when taking chasteberry, it may take several weeks to notice a significant decrease in hot flashes.

GINSENG (*PANAX GINSENG*)

Ginseng is known primarily for its ability to help the body overcome fatigue and stress, though its estrogen effect may aid in controlling hot flashes. Ginseng also acts to elevate your mood and acts as a rejuvenator.

Women with hypertension, heart problems, or clotting disorders should not take ginseng. While it will not cause these conditions to develop, it can aggravate these pre-existing conditions.

It is important to purchase your ginseng from a reputable source such as an herb or natural food store. Chinese pharmacies often have excellent selections. An herbologist also may be able to help you select a good-quality ginseng.

Available in several forms—tinctures, extracts, whole root, and powders—American and white/red Chinese ginseng root are the best. The suggested dose is two tablets twice a day, 1/4 teaspoon powder in warm water or tea three times a day, or 1/8 inch of whole root chewed daily.

LICORICE ROOT (*GLYCYRRHIZA GLABRA*)

Licorice has been recognized for centuries as an effective treatment for stomach ulcers, indigestion, respiratory problems, and because of its mild estrogenic effect, hot flashes. Licorice is one of the most widely prescribed herbs in China. It was also the favorite of the ancient Romans and Greeks, as well as the Germans and British. Hippocrates, the father of modern medicine, was known to prescribe the herb frequently. Caution should be exercised with high concentrations of this otherwise safe herb. High concentrations of glycyrheticinic acid found in licorice may cause sodium and water retention, possibly leading to a rise in blood pressure. Because of this, women with hypertension, kidney, and urinary tract problems should use licorice with caution and avoid extended use.

While phytoestrogens are safe in prescribed doses, it should be remembered that these substances exert an effect on your body chemistry and they must be respected. Just because a substance is "natural" doesn't mean that it can't have an adverse reaction in some people, or be harmful if taken in higher than normal doses. If you experience any ill effects or discomfort while using any of these herbs, discontinue their use immediately and consult your health care provider, herbalist, or nutritionist for further information.

NATURAL PROGESTERONE

Natural progesterone creams have received considerable attention recently. Used by Native Americans to relieve labor pains, they may also be helpful in relieving vaginal dryness and hot flashes.

Natural progesterone creams are made from a naturally occurring plant steroid called dioxgenin, found in wild yam roots (*Dioscorea villosa*). During the 1940s, Dr. Russell Marker used Mexican wild yams as his source of natural substances which can be chemically changed to create progestin, or norethindrone. This was the first progesterone used in birth control pills. It is important to note that wild yams were the source of raw material to make progesterone, not the progesterone itself. This point becomes particularly important when purchasing creams. Some claim to contain wild yam extract but fail to quantify the amount of progesterone it contains.

Quality progesterone creams are usually massaged into your skin. The thinner skin of the chest, breasts, lower abdomen, inner thighs, inner arms, wrist, and neck absorb the cream the best. It is also recommended that you rotate the application area.

Noticeable benefits may happen quickly or may take up to one to three months. For vaginal dryness, 1/4 to 1/2 teaspoon may be inserted into the vagina daily. For immediate relief, it may be used more than once a day. To control hot flashes, it is recommended you use 1/4 to 1/2 teaspoon every 15 minutes for the first hour following the episode, then 1/2 teaspoon once or twice a day for maintenance. More rapid benefits can be obtained by concurrent use of phytoestrogens.

A note of caution: It is extremely important to understand that there is only one FDA-approved cream available which gives a specific amount of natural progesterone with predictable blood levels. It is the only cream that should be used to balance estrogen replacement. It is called Crinone® and is a micronized progesterone cream. Other progesterone creams may not supply adequate levels of progesterone to protect the lining of the uterus from precancerous change.

Crinone® is supplied in prefilled vaginal applicators. It is rather costly but only needs to be used every other month to balance estrogen replacement. The initial recommended dose is 4 percent (45 mg) vaginally every other night for a total of 6 doses.

Possible side effects include:

▲ Fatigue

▲ Cramps

▲ Depression

▲ Headache

▲ Sleep disturbance

▲ Bloating

FAST FACTS
ALTERNATIVE THERAPIES

1. *Exercise*
   ▲ *Release of endorphins in hypothalamus*
   - *Controls body temperature*
   - *Relieves hot flashes*

2. *Diet*
   ▲ *Soybean products*
   - *Rich in phytoestrogens*
   - *One cup is equivalent in effect to 0.45 mg of conjugated estrogen (Premarin®).*

   ▲ *Fennel*
   - *High in phytoestrogens*
   - *TEA: 1 to 2 teaspoons of crushed seed to a cup of boiling water, steep for 10 minutes, drink 2 to 3 times a day*

   ▲ *High-lignan flaxseed oil*
   - *Felt to have protective effect against breast cancer*
   - *DOSAGE: one tablespoon daily*

   ▲ *Vitamin E*
   - *Women with high blood pressure, diabetes, rheumatic heart disease, or taking digitalis should consult health care provider before taking.*

   DOSAGE:
   - *800 IU daily until hot flashes subside, 400 IU daily thereafter*
   - *Take with B-complex vitamins, vitamin C (500 mg), selenium (25 mg)*

3. *Herbs*
   ▲ *Phytoestrogens*
   - *Two percent of the activity found in endogenous estrogen*
   - *Low-estrogen states provide estrogenic effect.*
   - *High-estrogen states bind to receptors and decrease estrogen's effect in body.*

- *Dong quai, licorice root, black cohosh, ginseng, and chasteberry are useful individually or in combination.*

▲ Dong quai
- *Popular in Asia for centuries*

DOSAGE
- *2 tablets, 2 times daily*
- *1/8 inch whole root eaten, 2 times daily*
- *1/4 teaspoon tincture mixed in tea or hot water, drink 2 times daily*

▲ Black Cohosh
- *Widely used by colonists, Native Americans, and now in Europe*

DOSAGE
- *Tablets containing 1 mg of 27-deoxyactein, 1 to 2 tablets twice daily or 2–4 mg/day*
- TEA: *1 teaspoon dried root in cup of water, boil, simmer for 10 minutes, drink 3 times a day*
- EXTRACT: *1 ml, 3 times a day*
- CAUTION: *Do not take if you have irregular heartbeat*

▲ Chasteberry
- *British women have used with success*

DOSAGE
- TEA: *pour 1 cup boiling water over 1 teaspoon fresh berries, steep for 10 minutes, drink 3 cups a day*
- EXTRACT: *1 ml, 3 times a day*

▲ Ginseng
- *Works as both a long-term rejuvenator and because of its estrogen effect, helps control hot flashes*

DOSAGE
- *2 tablets, 2 times a day*
- *1/4 teaspoon powder in warm water or tea, 2 times a day*

- *1/8 inch whole root chewed daily*
- *Purchase from reputable source*
- CAUTION: *Women with hypertension, heart disease, or clotting disorders should consult a health care provider before taking.*

▲ **Licorice Root**
- *Used for a variety of medical problems*
- *Dates back to Hippocrates*
- *Estrogen-like effect helpful with hot flashes*
- *Avoid high concentrations*
- *May cause water retention*
- *Women with hypertension, kidney, and urinary tract problems should use with caution.*

4. *Natural progesterone*

▲ *Useful for hot flashes and vaginal dryness*

▲ *Derived from wild yam root*

▲ *Be careful to purchase only creams that specify how much progesterone they contain.*

▲ *Apply to thinner skin of chest, breast, lower abdomen, inner thighs, inner arms, wrists, and neck.*
- *Rotate applications*

DOSAGE
- *Vaginal dryness*
  1/4 to 1/2 teaspoon inserted into vagina daily
- *Hot flashes*
  1/4 to 1/2 teaspoon every 15 minutes for first hour following episode, then 1/2 teaspoon once or twice daily
- *Concurrent use of phytoestrogens helps increase the effect.*
- CAUTION: *Until a method is available and approved by the FDA to deliver an adequate and effective dose of natural progesterone, it should not be used as the sole progestin to balance estrogen replacement therapy.*

6

Emotions and Moods

L et the truth be known. Studies have shown that there is no increased incidence of depression among perimenopausal women when compared to non-perimenopausal women. This is not to say that women don't become depressed. The incidence, however, is virtually the same for all women.

DEPRESSION

Where did women get the idea that they would suffer a major anxiety or depression episode while passing through perimenopause? The answer, I'm afraid, lies within the medical profession. One of the greatest injustices that the medical community has perpetuated for over a century was the concept of "Involutional Melancholia." Involutional refers to menopause. This term was used to describe a disorder thought to be common among menopausal women, characterized by worry, anxiety, agitation, and severe insomnia. Other symptoms noted were feelings of guilt and psychosomatic problems of delusional proportions.

Fortunately, in 1980, this term was finally removed from the American Psychiatric Association's "Diagnostic and Statistical Manual of Mental Disorders," which is considered to be the "bible" for mental health disorders. Unfortunately, it will take years before the legacy of this myth totally disappears from use.

While the stress women face during perimenopause may be unique to this period, the effect of the stress is virtually the same as any other age. Coping mechanisms remain intact and unaltered. If a perimenopausal woman does become depressed, it should not be assumed it is due to the changes her body is going through.

STRESS

Stressors unique to perimenopause may include being "sandwiched" between worrying about child care and the care of your own aging parents. Children leaving home or returning home with children of their own, dealing with chronic illness or death of a spouse, and financial concerns all add stress to a woman's life.

The good news is that there will also be relief from previous stress factors. Children may become more self-sufficient, leaving more time for you to pursue your own interests and career or to develop new ones. There is also freedom from the fear of pregnancy. Grandchildren often may be a blessing to help balance the new stressors. Perimenopause should be viewed as a new and exciting beginning, not an ending.

Empty nests do not need to be unhappy nests. A study in 1988 conducted by Northwestern University Medical Center used psychological tests to compare perimenopausal women with children at home to a group of women whose children were gone. Surprisingly, the women with the empty nests described themselves as more confident, independent, assertive, and goal-oriented. Those with children at home tended to be more submissive, nurturing, cautious, and dependent.

SLEEP DISTURBANCES

Sleep disturbances due to hot flashes with consequent chronic exhaustion may decrease a woman's coping mechanisms. This is the only unique change that truly affects the mood. What is important to realize is that correct treatment would be to control the nocturnal hot flashes, not simply take antidepressants or antianxiety medication, which may not be necessary.

PREMENSTRUAL SYNDROME (PMS)

Premenstrual syndrome may either increase in intensity or even appear for the first time during perimenopause. Irritability, anxiety, fatigue, and insomnia may appear in a cyclic fashion. It is often helpful to keep a symptoms journal (see the back of this book for a sample) to record what you are feeling and when it is occurring. This will aid in determining if symptoms are cycle-related or of a more general nature. If cyclic in nature, then they are most likely due to PMS.

Studies at PMS clinics have shown the following to be helpful in controlling your symptoms. To be effective, they should be started two weeks before you have your period.

Try these methods of treatment:

▲ Vitamin B$_6$, 50 to 100 mg per day, to decrease irritability.

▲ Vitamin E, 400 to 800 IU per day, to control breast tenderness.

▲ Avoid caffeine and chocolate to reduce both breast tenderness and irritability.

▲ Increase exercise, especially aerobic, to stimulate release of endorphins in your brain.

▲ Decrease salt intake to avoid water retention and swelling.

▲ Avoid concentrated sweets such as candy, items with sugar. Due to hormone changes in perimenopause, ingestion of sugar can be followed by a rapid fall in blood sugar.

▲ Add a multivitamin with iron.

▲ Add a calcium supplement.

Here are some general steps to relieve stress. Try the following and see if you don't feel better:

▲ Exercise regularly.

▲ Identify the sources of your stress. Write them down on one side of a sheet of paper; on the other side, list possible solutions. Don't be afraid to ask for help from a friend, spouse, or relative. Be creative.

▲ Pace yourself and start taking breaks. If being a caregiver contributes to your stress, don't be afraid to ask for help.

▲ Try relaxation techniques, including biofeedback and yoga.

  • Many self-help books are available which teach these skills.

  • Find a coach to help get started. Many times adult classes at your local high school or community college are good places to start.

▲ If things get out of control, don't delay, seek out a counselor. Therapy is usually limited to no more than 10 to 12 sessions and the rewards can be great.

MAJOR DEPRESSION

If you or someone you know is suffering from major depression, it is imperative to seek medical treatment immediately. The key difference between a major depressive episode and a case of the ordinary "blues" is the inability to perform your normal daily routine and responsibilities. Major depression overwhelms you and affects both your mind and body. Some people are predisposed genetically to developing depression. We may see a pattern developing within a family. Most times, however, there is no prior history of depression. Either way, the treatment is the same. Again, this is *not* more likely to occur during perimenopause than at any other age during your life.

Symptoms of major depression:

▲ Sleeping too much or too little.

▲ Inability to engage in previously pleasurable activities, such as the loss of sex drive

▲ Debility or loss of energy

▲ Feelings of worthlessness

▲ Difficulty concentrating, remembering, or making decisions

▲ Thoughts of committing suicide

▲ Eating too much or too little

GET HELP

Don't delay in getting help if you have any of these symptoms. Initially you will probably be started on an antidepressant medication to get you back into the mainstream. When your health care provider feels that you are strong enough for psychotherapy alone, medication is gradually withdrawn. Do not stop any medication before being instructed to no matter how good you may feel. You may just be feeling better because the medicine is doing its job.

It is important not to blame yourself for needing help. Depression is neither a character flaw nor a weakness. Twenty million adult Americans are affected each year by depression. One in eight individuals is affected over the course of their lifetime, although depression is twice as common in women than men.

Another reason not to delay seeking medical attention is to determine if your depression is truly psychological in origin. Many medical conditions such as thyroid disorders, diabetes, certain malignancies, infections, and neurologic problems can also present themselves as depression. Certain medications including some heart medications, hormones, and antibiotics, may also have a similar effect.

FAST FACTS
EMOTIONS AND MOODS

1. *No increase in the incidence of mental illness during perimenopause.*

2. *When it does occur, the picture is similar to younger and older ages.*

3. *Diagnosis of "Involutional Melancholia" has been discredited and abandoned.*

4. *Inability to cope may be due to exhaustion from sleep disturbances brought on by hot flashes rather than psychological problems.*

5. *PMS may either intensify or begin during perimenopause. Effective treatment is listed within this chapter.*

6. *Major depression requires immediate attention by a health care provider. There are many medical conditions that can also present as depression.*

Sexual Freedom

Contrary to what many women have been led to believe, your sex life does not end at perimenopause. Many women report that with freedom from the risk of pregnancy and with children grown, their sexual pleasure increased. This is supported by the results of all the large sexual research studies. The Kinsey report and Masters and Johnson both showed women can continue to enjoy sex well into old age, provided other health issues don't interfere.

INCREASED SEX DRIVE

Research has also shown that women can develop an increased sex drive during their late forties and early fifties. Both physical and social reasons cause this to occur. Physically, a higher testosterone to estrogen ratio exists (except in women who have had their ovaries removed). This is due to falling estrogen levels, not increases in testosterone. The testosterone is the dominant hormone found in men. However, it is responsible for libido or feelings of sexual desire in both sexes. Accompanying this relative increase in testosterone effect during perimenopause comes a greater sex drive.

Socially, with children grown, women can devote more time and energy on themselves. This includes their own sexual needs. Freedom from risk of pregnancy may lead to more spontaneity.

Women whose sexual interest fades and disappears during perimenopause are usually those who previously enjoyed it the least before. Menopause is used as an excuse to stop. If you find yourself in this group, know that it is never too late to rekindle old passions or develop new ones. A short course of counseling may be all that is necessary.

CHANGES IN SEXUAL STIMULATION

There will be some changes in the way your body responds to sexual stimulation. In this section, we will discuss these changes and show some simple adjustments that can be made to keep sex fun for you and your partner. Birth control options will also be reviewed for those still at risk for pregnancy. Most experts agree that the best way to avoid an unwanted pregnancy is to practice birth control for a full year following your last period.

What changes can you expect? With falling estrogen levels, the lining of the vagina becomes thinner and drier, making it less elastic. It will also become slightly shorter and narrower, although not too short or narrow to preclude sexual activity. The vulva also changes. The labia becomes smaller, thinner, and retracted, leading to greater exposure of the clitoris, which may be fairly sensitive to the touch. Adequate lubrication is the key element to keeping foreplay and intercourse enjoyable.

Your body will respond to stimulation differently than it did when you were younger. More stimulation is usually required to achieve adequate lubrication. Foreplay will need to be prolonged and you may find that adding a lubricant may be helpful. If the walls of the vagina are already thin and irritated, estrogen cream may also be necessary to achieve the desired results.

Vaginal dryness and irritation is probably the least discussed aspect of perimenopause, but represents a very real problem for many women. Fortunately, this can be treated easily and effectively.

When symptoms are not severe, nonhormonal treatments should be tried first.

▲ Water-soluble lubricating gels can be applied to the outside of the vagina and a small amount inside as well. You can apply some to your partner's penis, making it part of your foreplay. Water-soluble gels are preferred since they are less likely to cause infection and do not stain clothing or bedsheets. They can also easily be washed off. Petroleum gel is not slippery enough and should not be used.

▲ Vaginal moisturizers, currently available over-the-counter, were designed to replenish vaginal moisture when used on a regular basis. Lubricants are inserted into the vagina by an applicator two to three times a week.

▲ Vitamin E vaginal suppositories have been found to be very effective by many naturopaths. The usual dose is nightly for six weeks, then switching to a weekly schedule.

▲ It is also helpful to prolong foreplay, giving your body some additional time to respond and self-lubricate. Having your partner use some water-soluble gel on his fingers will also be helpful to help lubricate your body.

▲ Some studies have shown that regular sexual activity either with your partner or through masturbation helps to keep the vagina lubricated. The exact reason is unclear, but greater blood flow to the area with regular stimulation has been suggested.

▲ Avoid douches, bubble bath, and perfumed bath oils. They all dry and irritate the vulva and vagina, resulting in dryness and itchiness.

ESTROGEN CREAM

When local lubricants no longer offer satisfactory results you may want to consider estrogen vaginal cream. Estrogen cream is helpful even if you are already using estrogen orally or through a patch. While estrogen pills and patches offer some relief, it may not be enough. Rather than increase the estrogen dose for the entire body, it is more efficient and safer to apply it only directly where needed. Estrogen cream can also be helpful for women with a history of breast cancer or other medical conditions where internal hormone replacement treatment is not advisable.

Initially there may be some absorption into the bloodstream, causing some breast tenderness. As the vaginal walls return to their normal thickness, only small amounts are absorbed into the bloodstream and breast tenderness resolves itself.

The usual dose is 1/2 applicator (1 gram) every other night for two to four weeks or until symptoms subside, then decrease the usage to two times a week. If you are going to have intercourse on a treatment night, the cream should be inserted after intercourse.

Your partner may also be experiencing some changes in his body. Men require more time to obtain an erection as they age, several minutes rather than seconds. Ejaculation may take longer to achieve and is less forceful and shorter in duration. This may actually be used to heighten your and your partner's pleasure, since premature ejaculation usually is no longer a problem. Men will also lose their erection quicker after orgasm as they get older. Their refractory period, the length of time after an erection and before another is possible, will increase. This will increase from the several minutes it takes in their twenties, to several hours in their forties and fifties, to several days when they reach their seventies and after.

These changes need not be a problem if you both recognize them, discuss them, and work together to make any necessary adjustments. Finding the right moment to bring up these issues is very important. Men don't always verbalize their fears of impotence when they first notice these changes. Reassurance is usually all that is necessary, but suggest they check with their health care provider to make sure there isn't an underlying medical condition.

TESTOSTERONE DILEMMA

Articles are beginning to appear supporting the addition of testosterone to hormone replacement therapy. This was prompted by claims of increased libido and renewed self-confidence when using testosterone. It should be noted that these claims are controversial, and taking testosterone is not without potential side effects.

Testosterone is the primary male sex hormone. It is responsible for their muscular physique, development of facial hair, deepening of their voice, and in some situations, an increase in aggressive behavior. Women also produce this hormone, but only at 1/10 of the amount as a man. In both sexes, testosterone appears to influence the limbic system, in turn causing an increase in sexual desire.

The studies quoted in support of adding testosterone have been principally conducted on women who have had a surgical menopause, which is the removal of ovaries. In women, testosterone is primarily produced in the ovaries and to a lesser extent, by the adrenal glands. Since the women in the studies had surgically lost their primary source of testosterone, it would seem reasonable that oral replacement of testosterone would be beneficial. The question is if it truly benefits a woman whose ovaries are intact and whose testosterone level is currently normal. Certainly more research is needed to answer this question.

While clinical studies do not clearly define the role of supplemental testosterone in women with intact ovaries, there is a growing body of testimonials supporting its use as well as support from the world literature.

Indeed, there are several well-researched and well-written books which draw on the world literature to support testosterone supplementation. Blood tests for testosterone measure both total and free (active) testosterone. These tests can determine if a deficiency exists.

It should be noted that methyltestosterone, the form found in the most commonly prescribed form of testosterone supplement, cannot be measured by standard tests for total testosterone. Its presence will be reflected in the free form. Therefore, in order to obtain an accurate measurement of total and free testosterone the woman should not be taking methyltestosterone. Natural testosterone does not have this problem.

There are advantages and disadvantages to using methyltestosterone. The advantage is it is not converted easily to estrogen, which is true with natural testosterone. This avoids the potential cancer risks from extremely high estrogen levels. The main disadvantage is that long-term use can lead to liver toxicity. Currently methyltestosterone is usually prescribed combined with estrogen in a single tablet. The dose is fixed and may be much higher than necessary. Although it requires the use of a compounding pharmacist, methyltestosterone pills can be made to order in various dosages.

Natural micronized testosterone is usually mixed with petrolatum jelly and available from a compounding pharmacist in

1 percent, 1 1/2 percent, and 2 percent concentrations. It is best to start at a lower dose and increase only as necessary to avoid very high blood levels.

The jelly is applied directly to the vulva (use no more than 1/4 teaspoon) every night. Blood levels should be checked after sixty days. As your levels return to normal decrease your use to three to four times a week. Blood levels should then be checked periodically and the dose adjusted to maintain normal range. Very high doses should be avoided to prevent adverse effects on the liver and blood cholesterol and potential masculinizing effects.

Topical testosterone cream can lose its potency after several months. It is best prepared in small quantities (usually no more than a three-month supply).

It is also important to be honest in deciding if your decreased libido could really be a sign of underlying depression. On the other hand, if you have enjoyed a healthy sexual desire that has now disappeared, but have no other signs of depression, testosterone may be beneficial.

Side Effects

Potential side effects of taking excessive testosterone include an adverse effect on your lipid profile (decreasing HDL or "good cholesterol"), possibly increasing your risk for cardiovascular diseases, and masculinizing effects, such as increased facial and body hair, acne, and oily skin. Certainly, it is important to gather information and discuss with your health care provider all aspects of this issue before taking testosterone.

BIRTH CONTROL

Most experts agree that in order to avoid an unwanted pregnancy, some form of birth control should be practiced for one full year following your last period. Although fertility rates decrease for women after age forty, ovulation still occurs and pregnancy is still a possibility even in spite of missed periods. However, an FSH level greater than 50 ensures that your chance of conceiving is almost nonexistent.

Selecting the best birth control method for your forties and into your fifties will require taking other changes into consideration.

For women having irregular or heavy periods with or without PMS, one of the new ultra-low estrogen pills (20 mcg estrogen) may be extremely helpful. In the same patient, an IUD may only aggravate the bleeding. An IUD, however, may be quite appropriate for a woman with normal periods who doesn't want to take birth control pills.

Birth Control Pills

Previously, women were discouraged from taking birth control pills after the age of forty, or after the age of thirty-five if they smoked. The 20 mcg pills now available have recently caused changes to be made to this recommendation. With the lack of cardiovascular risk, these pills can be used safely by a nonsmoker until menopause. Smokers need to be counseled on an individual basis to determine appropriate use of birth control. The advantages of pill use are cycle regulation, with decreases in cramping and bleeding, protection from both endometrial (uterine) and ovarian cancers, and relief from hot flashes. The protection against endometrial and ovarian cancer continues five to ten years after the pills have been discontinued, if they were taken for at least five years. Contrary to some beliefs, the pill will not delay or accelerate your menopause. A commonly asked question is, "How will I know when I pass through menopause if I'm on the pill?" The answer is, you won't know until you discontinue their use. At that point, you can decide between hormone replacement therapy or alternative treatments.

Intrauterine Device (IUD)

The IUD being marketed today can be left in place for eight to ten years without problems. Some years ago, they were withdrawn from the market because of the potential risk of pelvic inflammatory disease in young non-monogamous women. Pelvic inflammation disease can in turn lead to infertility. For a monogamous woman who has finished her childbearing and has a regular period, the IUD can work quite well.

If you do decide to use an IUD, it is important to report any changes in your bleeding pattern. Fever, chills, and lower abdominal pain with or without a vaginal discharge should also be brought to your health care provider's attention immediately.

Barrier Methods—Diaphragm, Condoms, Foam, and Cervical Cap

Since women in their forties and fifties are more knowledgeable about their bodies and often have a higher motivation not to get pregnant, these methods are quite useful and effective for this age group. A diaphragm, when used properly, can be over 95 percent effective. The combination of condoms and contraceptive gel, foam, or suppositories, is over 90 percent reliable. Possible drawbacks include irritation from the contraceptive gel and difficulty in correctly placing a diaphragm if vaginal or uterine prolapse exists. Because the diaphragm sits behind the pubic bone in the front and the upper vagina in the back, improper placement and use has been associated with recurrent urinary tract infections caused by inadequate emptying of the bladder, especially after intercourse.

Sterilization

Close to 100 percent effective, sterilization is safe and easy to perform. The question is which partner should undergo the procedure.

Vasectomy

Vasectomy is an office-based procedure, requiring only local anesthesia and mild sedation. Quick and easy to perform by a qualified physician, some techniques don't even require external sutures. The recovery is usually quick and often a man is able to return to normal activities in a day or two, wearing scrotal support.

Tubal Ligation

Tubal ligation is an outpatient procedure. However, it does require general anesthesia, where most of the risk lies. In both the vasectomy and tubal ligation, the tubes (vas deferens in men and fallopian tubes in women) are either tied and cut, clipped and cut, or cauterized to prevent passage of sperm or eggs. Other potential problems associated with laparoscopic tubal ligation include puncture of a major blood vessel or an internal organ such as the bowel, while inserting the instruments through the abdominal wall. While rare, this may occur even in the most experienced of hands.

Both procedures should be considered permanent and irreversible. While reversal surgery is available for both procedures, it is quite expensive and there are no guarantees that it will be successful. In-vitro fertilization (IVF) and sperm-retrieval procedures are also available for couples desiring a child. But these procedures are expensive and not generally covered by an insurance plan. It is best, however, to be as certain as possible that you do not and will never want additional children before you or your partner undergo any sterilization procedure.

Natural Family Planning

Natural family planning is based on the principle that a woman usually ovulates fourteen days prior to her menses (period). By keeping a calendar record and/or by testing her own cervical mucus (it changes at the time of ovulation), a woman with a regular, consistent cycle will be able to predict when she should ovulate and avoid intercourse at these times.

As I have previously mentioned, ovulation may occur erratically and cervical mucus, which can indicate when you are fertile, may be minimal during perimenopause. So there are fewer signs to alert you to ovulation. Because of these changes in ovulatory frequency and menstrual patterns, natural methods are less reliable during this period.

FAST FACTS
SEXUAL FREEDOM

1. *Perimenopause has been shown to be a time when women not only continue to enjoy sex, but their libido and satisfaction may be heightened.*

2. *There will be some changes in the way your body responds to sexual stimulation.*

   ▲ *A decrease in lubrication may require some intervention.*

   ▲ *Longer foreplay*

   ▲ *Vaginal, water-soluble lubricants, moisturizers, or vitamin E suppositories*

   ▲ *If associated with significant drying, use vaginal estrogen or natural progesterone cream.*

   ▲ *Avoid douches, bubble baths, perfumed bath oils.*

3. *Your partner will also experience some changes in his sexual response.*

   ▲ *Longer time to obtain an erection*
   - *Minutes rather than seconds*

   ▲ *Ejaculation may take longer to achieve.*
   - *This may be a benefit as there may be less premature ejaculations.*

   ▲ *Longer refractory period*
   - *Hours between erections in their forties and fifties, rather than minutes as in their twenties.*
   - *Reassurance may be necessary that these changes are normal and not signs of impotence.*

4. *Adding testosterone to hormone replacement therapy*

   ▲ *Claims that it can increase libido and self-confidence*

   ▲ *Studies were done on women who have had their ovaries surgically removed.*

   ▲ *Normally testosterone levels remain constant throughout a woman's life, as long as her ovaries and adrenal glands are intact.*

▲ It's important to determine if decreased libido is due to hormonal change or a sign of depression.

▲ Potential problems
  • Adverse effect on lipid profile
  • Masculinizing changes

5. Birth Control

▲ To avoid unwanted pregnancy, practice birth control one full year following last period, unless FSH blood level is greater than 50.

▲ Birth control pills
  • Effective very low dose 20 mcg estrogen pills now available
  • Helpful for women with irregular cycles or heavy flows
  • Relieves PMS symptoms
  • Controls hot flashes and vaginal dryness
  • Protection against uterine and ovarian cancer

6. IUD

▲ Effective long-term use

▲ May remain in place for eight to ten years

▲ Monogamous relationship to avoid infection

▲ Not good choice for women with heavy or irregular menses

7. Barrier Methods

▲ Diaphragm, condoms and foam, cervical cap

▲ Quite useful for women in their forties and fifties who are knowledgeable about their bodies

▲ High motivation required

▲ Potential problems
  • Poor fitting of diaphragm in women with uterine or bladder prolapse.
  • Recurrent urinary tract infection with poorly fitted diaphragm.

8. *Sterilization*

▲ *Vasectomy*
- *Local anesthesia*
- *Office procedure*
- *Minimal recovery time*
- *Few complications*

▲ *Tubal Ligation (Laparoscopic)*
- *General anesthesia*
- *Out-patient surgical procedure*
- *Rare but potential complications of major bleeding or puncture of bowel*
- *Recovery of two to three days*

9. *Natural Family Planning*

▲ *Not a good choice in this age group*
- *Ovulation occurs irregularly.*
- *Decreased cervical mucus*

Exercise the Mind and Body

The importance of initiating and then continuing an exercise program can't be overstated. If anyone is looking for a "fountain of youth," this is the closest you'll get. Exercise provides a way to take control of the aging process while literally slowing it down. It increases your energy level, makes you more alert, prevents heart disease, lowers your blood pressure, raises the levels of HDL (good) cholesterol, and strengthens your bones to help prevent osteoporosis. By increasing the release of endorphins, which are your body's natural tranquilizer, exercise has an overall calming effect on your mood. In fact, studies have shown that regular exercise may be as effective as psychotherapy for treating mild to moderate depression.

With a better self-image, exercise promotes a positive attitude, greater creativity, and a feeling of being in control of your life. And it is never too late to begin. So let's take a look at the basic principles of exercise, discuss the different types, and design a program best suited to your needs.

SCIENTIFIC BACKGROUND

A little scientific background is in order first. Contrary to what is popularly believed, your body does not completely stop making estrogen after menopause. What changes is the mechanism of production and the levels attained. After menopause, your adrenal glands, one located over each kidney, together with the ovaries produce the hormone androsteindione. This hormone is circulated by the bloodstream to all the fat cells of the body where it is then converted to estrogen. The liver and kidneys also aid in this conversion. This supply of estrogen can ease the physical signs of perimenopause. The amount of estrogen produced in this way varies with each woman. The exciting news is that exercise stimulates the adrenal glands to increase androseindione production which ultimately leads to an increase in estrogen. In this way, exercise has a direct effect on decreasing hot flashes, vaginal dryness, and osteoporosis. Since the adrenal glands are the major source of androsteindione, it's important to keep them healthy. The best way to keep adrenal glands healthy is to avoid caffeine, concentrated sugars, and to keep alcohol to a minimum. All of these cause stress to the adrenal glands. The B-complex vitamins and vitamin C are also helpful in keeping the adrenals stress-free.

AN OUNCE OF PREVENTION

Preventing osteoporosis requires two things, both exercise and increasing dietary calcium. The earlier you begin, the more successful your efforts will be. Weight-bearing exercise is the best. Some excellent weight-bearing exercises include:

▲ Walking

▲ Running

▲ Aerobic dance

▲ Cross-country skiing

Swimming and rowing, although not technically weight-bearing exercises, have also been shown to be effective. These two are especially helpful for someone with previous hip, knee, or ankle injury, in a woman who is overweight, or who may suffer from arthritis.

A two-year study, conducted by the Washington University School of Medicine in St. Louis, looked at women, ages fifty-five to seventy, and compared those who engaged in regular exercise programs and took 1500 mg of calcium a day to a control group, who took only calcium. At the end of the study, bone density scans revealed a 61 percent increase in bone mass in the exercise group and a 1 percent loss of bone mass in the control group who didn't exercise.

The Nurses Study referred to earlier in our discussion of HRT also found that regular exercise reduced the risk of heart disease as much as 40 percent. This can be achieved by walking at a brisk pace for 30 to 45 minutes, three times a week .

CHANGES IN METABOLISM

Two interesting changes take place regarding our metabolism after age thirty-five. First, it slows sufficiently that we begin to gain weight not by eating more but by eating the same amount. Secondly, it takes on characteristics from our ancestral tradition to hunt and gather. This simply means that if we try to lose weight by only decreasing our intake of calories, our metabolism slows down proportionally. Certainly this served as an important survival technique helping to conserve fat stores when food was scarce. Today, however, this is nothing but a nuisance. With this in mind, you can see that when you start a diet, you experience an initial period of rapid weight loss, which is quickly followed by a slowing of weight loss and eventual plateau. You may find yourself trying as hard as you can to lose weight and you are just not losing any. This is when many people become frustrated and give up and no wonder. Another failed diet.

COMBAT THOSE CHANGES

The key is to add exercise, which speeds up your metabolism. By speeding up your metabolism, you burn the extra stored calories in the form of unwanted fat. Not only do you burn fat while you are exercising, but research has shown we continue to burn it at a faster rate for hours after you stop exercising. Exercise also helps stabilize your blood sugar, aiding in the prevention and control of diabetes. Increased circulation to the skin gives you better color and stimulates the production of collagen. This is the protein which makes skin more pliable and retards wrinkles. Libido may also be given a boost by exercising. By easing your stress, interest may be renewed. You are also more fit and have an improved body image, which may be helpful also.

People often confuse an active life with exercising. Running around doing errands or being on your feet all day may make you tired, but usually this is more because of a mental exhaustion rather than physical exhaustion. There are multiple studies that show that the benefits are not the same as those derived from dedicated physical exercise.

BEFORE YOU START

Consult your health care provider if you are over thirty-five, have been sedentary, or have a past history of hypertension, diabetes, heart disease, or any other medical condition that might require special attention. Even if you have no prior history of heart problems—if you are out of shape, you should have a complete physical, including an evaluation of your blood pressure and an EKG. Hypertension and some heart problems may be difficult to detect in sedentary people. It's not until they exert themselves that these conditions are revealed, sometimes with disastrous results. Your health care provider may also recommend a cardiac stress test. This involves being connected to an EKG machine, while walking on a treadmill. By progressively increasing the incline of the treadmill, greater degrees of stress are placed on the heart. This is continued until your maximum heart rate is reached. An ultrasound of your heart can also be done at this time, called an echocardiogram. This allows the cardiologist to evaluate the heart's valves, wall motion, and output. The EKG during this test would show signs of any irregularities in the rate or rhythm of the heart, decreased blood and oxygen supply to the heart itself, or any blocks or alterations in the electrical signals in the heart.

GETTING STARTED

Once you have been cleared to exercise, it is important to design a program that works the entire body and fits into your schedule. It should include exercises that increase flexibility, endurance, and strength. This means stretching, aerobic, and weight-training exercises. Few single exercises offer all three. Running, for example, is a great aerobic exercise which builds cardiovascular endurance and strength in the lower extremities. Unfortunately, it does nothing for upper-body strength or overall flexibility. Your exercise program should either require you to continue exercise, like running while swinging light weights, or better yet develop a routine of several activities such as weight training, stationary bike, and stretching.

CUSTOMIZE YOUR PLAN

The single most important concept when designing your exercise program is to make it as convenient, inexpensive, and easy to perform as possible. Doing this will help to ensure your long-term success. If you must get into your car, drive 20 minutes to a health club, change your clothes, exercise, shower, and change again—how long do you think you'll realistically continue it? The truth is not very long at all. In fact the entire health club industry gets rich on just that principle.

It's best to design your exercise program around a primary exercise that builds cardiovascular fitness. You then add strengthening and flexibility exercises. Remember, keep it simple, just walk out your front door to walk briskly or run. Keep it inexpensive, all you need are a good pair of supportive walking or running shoes, a set of light dumbbells or resistance bands. Easy to perform, there are many great exercise books that explain individual strengthening and flexibility exercise. Your public library or local bookstore will probably have several good books to choose from.

AEROBIC EXERCISE

What is aerobic exercise? Aerobic means oxygen. Aerobic exercises cause you to breathe in more air and make the heart work faster and harder in order to circulate the oxygen throughout your body. In order for this type of exercise to be beneficial, it is necessary to maintain a certain level of intensity for 20 to 30 minutes at least three times a week. The level of activity is determined by calculating your target pulse rate.

For those who have never checked their pulse, it is a fairly simple procedure. The two most convenient locations are the carotid arteries in your neck and the radial artery in your wrist. Personally, I prefer the carotid artery, especially after exercising. It is easier to find, being more pronounced. Practice taking your pulse while sitting quietly. Use the first two fingers of either hand and start working your way across your neck, just under your jaw. Move from outside, toward your windpipe. About halfway, you will feel a strong pulse. This is the carotid artery. Now count the beats for 10 seconds and multiply that number by 6. You now know your "resting pulse."

Next, determine your training heart rate. To do this, you must first determine your "maximum heart rate." Take 200, subtract your age, then multiply your answer, the estimated maximum heart rate, by 0.7 and 0.85. This will give you the lower and upper range of your training heart rate. Here is an example:

$200 - 45$ years old	$=$	155 is your maximum heart rate
155×0.7	$=$	109 is your lower training heart rate
155×0.85	$=$	135 is your upper training heart rate

Use the space provided in "Fast Facts" at the end of the chapter to calculate your range.

If you have been sedentary, start slowly and gradually, over several months, working up to the 70 percent range. Not only is it dangerous to overextend yourself, but you will burn out quickly, possibly become discouraged, and quit. Remember, every day you exercise, no matter how slowly, is better than no exercise at all. Even if you are unable to see the changes, they are taking place inside your body. Every day you exercise—you are getting stronger and more healthy.

Do all the calculations seem too complicated? There is a way of estimating if you are exercising within your target heart range. Studies have shown that if you can just about keep up a conversation without gasping while exercising, you are quite close to your training range.

Varying the intensity of your aerobic workout is also important. In general, the faster heart rates are better for cardiovascular conditioning. To burn fat, you want your pace slower and your workout longer. For example, an hour of brisk walking at a pulse rate of 120 burns more fat than 20 minutes of running at a pulse rate of 150.

To avoid boredom and to help prevent plateaus, it is best to "cross train." This means alternating your aerobic exercise. For example, you could switch off between rowing, treadmill or power walking, swimming, running, and aerobic dance.

WALKING

Walking fits all the criteria of good exercise. It's convenient, inexpensive, easy to perform, relieves tension and anxiety, and improves circulation. A mile of walking burns as many calories as a mile of running, it just takes longer. It should be accompanied by brisk arm swinging. One- to two-pound dumbbells may also be carried in each hand. Try to work up to a pace of 15 minutes per mile, and remember, you need to supplement walking with both upper-body stretching and flexibility exercises.

RUNNING

Running also satisfies the three criteria for good exercise. It gets you in shape faster, but you should start by alternating running with walking. You should also supplement running with upper-body strengthening and flexibility exercises. Be sure to wear a good pair of supportive, cushioning running shoes. They may cost a little extra, but may save you from eventual knee and ankle injury. It is also recommended that you replace your athletic shoes every 3 to 6 months, depending on the intensity of your training program, or as soon as you feel a decrease in their cushioning capacity.

SWIMMING

Swimming is probably one of the best all-around exercises. It combines strengthening, endurance, and flexibility. It is also quite useful for someone with arthritis or joint injury as it cushions the impact of the exercise on the joints. While swimming is not a weight-bearing exercise, some research shows an increase in bone density among swimmers. Obviously, you will need access to a pool. This need not be expensive, try your local YWCA or community center. Just be sure the pool is convenient enough so you will stick to your program.

ROWING

Rowing is an excellent all-around exercise that provides strengthening, endurance, and flexibility with a full range of motion of all the major muscle groups. It does require access to a rowing machine or a nice straight stretch of water. The best machine is called an ergometer, which was designed by rowers for rowers to imitate the fluid movement of a boat. It's a little more costly, but worth the investment, especially since you can start at any age and continue forever. The machines are available from many sport retail stores or can even be ordered factory direct. You may want to avoid the piston-type rowing machine which is more rigid and does not allow for the same flow of movement. While less expensive, they don't offer the same rewards.

AEROBIC DANCE

Depending on your level of motivation, you can either purchase a videotape for home use or join a class. When choosing a videotape, choose one that will keep your interest and maintain your enthusiasm. You will find a large, diverse selection of videotapes on the market. Many of the health clubs in your area may offer aerobic classes, just remember to make sure you choose one that is convenient. A good pair of supportive athletic shoes is necessary; ask your dance instructor or personal trainer/coach which shoe is right for you.

CROSS-COUNTRY SKIING

While not the least expensive or most convenient unless you live in a snowy climate, cross-country skiing is probably the most fun and a great all-around exercise. A good alternative is a cross-country ski machine which offers the same aerobic benefits and range of motion as hitting the trails outdoors. It can be done in your own home during any season.

WEIGHT TRAINING

A weight training program is divided into two basic functions. The first is "reps," which is short for repetition. A rep is one complete movement up or down, back and forth. Completion of a rep means returning to the starting position. The second is "set." A set includes a fixed number of reps.

How much weight should you start lifting? You should use enough weight so that you can complete the prescribed number of reps, but the last rep should feel difficult. When the last rep feels too easy, you know it's time to add more weight.

How many reps should you do? Perform a particular exercise until you feel a slight burning in the muscle group being worked. Ten reps per set is a fairly standard amount. If you can do more than ten reps before feeling the burning sensation, then you need to increase the weight.

Never jerk or twist the weights. The slower you perform a rep, the greater the benefit. Muscle fibers strengthen in proportion to the length of time they are stressed. The longer you keep them stressed, the greater the benefit. Each part of the exercise should take the same amount of time. This is called passive resistance and strength is increased faster using this method.

Never exercise the same muscle groups two days in a row. Alternate the upper body one day, then the lower body weight exercises the next day. Muscles require 24 to 48 hours to recover and grow. Another option would be to alternate weight training one day with aerobic exercise the next.

Dumbbells are probably the best all-around weights. They are relatively inexpensive and easy to store. Their greatest advantages are they offer a broader range of movement and you don't need a spotter—someone to assist you to avoid injury—when working out. While barbells can only be moved in one direction at a time, dumbbells can be rotated through a full range. There are some excellent books that demonstrate the flexibility of using dumbbells.

If you are worrying about developing bulging muscles from lifting weights, don't be. Women do not generally have high enough testosterone levels to cause that to happen. Testosterone is the primary male hormone and responsible for a masculine physique. For women, weight training will simply add better definition of your normal feminine shape.

Increasing bone density should be your primary concern. When muscles contract during weight training, they stimulate the bone underneath to conserve calcium. This in turn produces denser and stronger bones.

STRETCH

Don't forget to stretch. Of all the other types of exercises, this is the most important. Unfortunately it is most often the one most neglected. Its purpose is to prevent injuries during your exercise routine. Stretching is mistakenly viewed as not being "real" exercise. With the time constraints we all have, we many times opt to jump right into something more strenuous, trying to gain the most from the little time we have. This can have painful long-term consequences. By not loosening up the muscles, tendons, and ligaments before you exercise, you can over-stress not only these structures but joints as well. Not stretching may result in torn muscle attachments, fractures, and permanent damage to the cartilage in joints.

Stiffness comes from the forming of cross-links or bridges between muscle fibers. These can form virtually overnight, which is why we many times complain of being stiff in the morning. These bridges become thicker and more numerous with time. Joint and muscle movement gradually becomes more and more restricted during sedentary periods. You can understand why that happens unless these bridges are broken up by stretching. A ligament, muscle, or joint may give out first.

Stretching should not hurt. You want to move in a certain direction until you feel a mild tension, then back off a little and hold it in place for 5 to 15 seconds. Never bounce or force a stretch. A stretch should feel like you can hold it forever. Pushing a stretch too far can cause microscopic tears in the muscle fibers. Scarring results with a gradual loss of elasticity. Give it time and be patient. Yoga, aerobic dance, and Tai Chi are all good ways to stretch while increasing flexibility. There are books on stretching, so check your library or favorite bookstore for the latest selections.

Don't forget your abdominals. No one likes to do sit-ups, but strengthening your abdominal muscles not only tones up your tummy but prevents lower back strain while also improving bladder control. The old straight leg sit-ups where you pulled yourself all the way up have been replaced. They were abandoned because it was found that they actually strained the lower back. The new method is called a modified crunch. With your knees bent, you lift only your shoulders off the floor. With this method, there is no back strain and results are as good as, if not better. You will also need to do leg lifts and lateral abdominal exercises to round out your workout. Lateral abdominal exercises are done in the basic sit-up position with your knees bent. Rather than lift your shoulders straight up, turn as you lift to face one or the other knee. This rotation movement exercises the muscles on either side of your abdomen, called the transverse abdominals. There are several instructional videos available. Start with a basic routine and advance at your own pace.

Personal Trainers

Personal trainers have recently become extremely popular. While more costly, they can be quite helpful, especially for someone who has been sedentary for some time or who has never exercised before. By showing you the correct way to exercise and helping you design your own program, you may find just a few sessions to be invaluable. You may want to try your local YWCA or community center first. At some clubs you can share a trainer with other clients, splitting the cost of the personal trainer.

Sample Schedule

Start strengthening and flexibility exercises 10 to 15 minutes every day. Do your aerobic exercises 20 to 30 minutes a day, 3 to 4 times a week. Start slow and build up to your target heart rate. Remember to cool down by gradually slowing down over 3 to 5 minutes. Never stop abruptly! Strengthening exercises should be done for 30 minutes a day, 3 times a week. Alternate these with aerobic exercises.

Track Your Progress

Keep a journal of your progress. Remember to be realistic about your goals. Be patient—it may take 6 weeks or more before you notice any results. Also expect some soreness in the beginning. Your muscles may not have worked this hard in years, but they will love you for it in the end. However, stop exercising immediately if you feel short of breath, experience muscle pain, chest pain, numbness, or become lightheaded. If these symptoms don't subside within a few minutes of rest, call your health care provider.

Buddy Up

Find a friend or acquaintance to exercise with. You will keep each other on track and prevent inertia from taking over. Everyone starts with good intentions, but staying with a program in spite of boredom, plateaus, or a million other reasons, is really the key to long-term success.

Keep yourself well hydrated. Drink eight ounces of water before and eight ounces of water after you exercise. Avoid alcohol and caffeinated beverages after exercising. Both act as diuretics and may cause you to become dehydrated.

Try to develop a certain "exercise consciousness." Look for ways to increase your exercise throughout the day, not simply limiting yourself to "official" workouts. For example—start taking stairs instead of elevators. If you're able to, go for a brisk walk at lunch or on breaks. Keep a small rubber ball in your desk drawer and squeeze it while talking on the phone or reading.

On your day off the exercise schedule, spend some time noticing the benefits of your training. You'll have more energy, a better self-image, and a stronger sense of well-being.

FAST FACTS

EXERCISE THE MIND AND BODY

1. *Think of exercise as your "fountain of youth." It increases energy levels and alertness, lowers blood pressure, prevents heart disease, strengthens bones, and has a calming effect on mood.*

2. **Dieting alone is ineffective, due to changes that occur in your metabolism as you get older.** *You need exercise to burn off extra calories.*

3. **Before you begin, see your health care provider and have a complete physical examination.** *Be sure to have your blood pressure evaluated and an EKG. You may need a cardiac stress test as well.*

4. **Design a program that is convenient, inexpensive, and easy to perform.**

5. **To get off on the right foot, consider a few sessions with a personal trainer or a good coach.**

6. **Take your pulse and calculate your maximum heart rate and your upper and lower training rates.**

   200 – Your age _____ = Maximum heart rate _____
   Maximum heart rate _____ x 0.7 = Lower training rate _____
   Maximum heart rate _____ x 0.85 = Upper training rate _____

7. **Develop a program that includes aerobic, weight-bearing, and flexibility exercises.**

8. **Don't forget to stretch before and after exercising.**

9. **"Cross train."** *To decrease boredom and avoid plateaus, alternate several aerobic exercises:*
   - ▲ *Walking*
   - ▲ *Running*
   - ▲ *Swimming*
   - ▲ *Rowing*
   - ▲ *Aerobic dance*

10. **Weight training**
    ▲ *Dumbbells work best.*
    ▲ *Never jerk or twist the weights.*
    ▲ *Perform each rep slowly. Take the same amount of time on extension as returning back to the starting position.*
    ▲ *Avoid exercising the same muscle groups two days in a row.*

11. **Sample schedule**
    ▲ *Stretch/flexibility exercises, 10 to 15 minutes a day*
    ▲ *Aerobic exercises:*
      • *Warm up 2 to 3 minutes.*
      • *20 to 30 minutes at training heart rate*
      • *Cool down 2 to 3 minutes.*
      • *Never stop abruptly!*
      • *3 to 4 days a week*
    ▲ *Strengthening exercises:*
      • *30 minutes, 3 days a week*
      • *Alternate with aerobic workouts*

12. **Remember to keep a journal of your exercise progress.**
    ▲ *Record your initial blood pressure pulse and weight at the start of your program.*
    ▲ *Record this data every month to monitor your progress.*

13. **Keep in mind that muscle weighs more than fat.** As you build muscle, your weight may stabilize or even climb a little, but notice how well your clothes fit.

14. **Stop exercising immediately if you feel short of breath, experience chest pains, muscle pain, numbness, or become lightheaded.** Call your health care provider if the symptoms don't subside within a few minutes of rest.

15. **Drink lots of water.** Avoid alcohol or caffeinated drinks after exercising due to their diuretic effect and the risk of dehydration.

Eating to Stay Fit

A sound diet is essential to good health. There is no way around it. The good news is, it doesn't have to be painful. As long as you form a solid foundation, you can enjoy treats—in moderation. Moderation is the key word, not total denial. Denial doesn't work in the long run, and it is the quickest way to condemn a diet to failure.

REWARDS OF HEALTHY FOOD

The rewards of healthy eating are many. Increasing the body's defense against chronic illness (heart disease, cancer, arthritis, and diabetes), and slowing the aging process by providing a greater reserve of nutrients for cell and tissue to remain strong, are just two of the many reasons to eat right. However, you must make it a way of life.

This chapter will review the individual components of good nutrition. We'll discuss how to structure your own food plan with methods for losing weight and keeping it off. Also, we will review why most diets fail and show you how to avoid these common pitfalls.

Rather than starting with the four major food groups, let's take it one step further and break them down into the main nutrition groups. These nutrition groups include protein, carbohydrates, fat, water, vitamins, and minerals. Understanding these important building blocks leads to a greater understanding of how to use each one to customize a food plan to your own individual tastes.

PROTEIN

Proteins should comprise 15 percent of our total caloric intake. The key is to obtain more proteins from vegetables and less from animal sources. The fat content of meat is the reason for this change. Surprisingly, most Americans eat 2 to 4 times more protein than they need. Unfortunately, most of it comes from animal sources, including eggs, meat, poultry, fish, and dairy products. Our high protein diet also promotes the loss of calcium in the urine. Long-term, this may help to accelerate bone loss.

Red meat should be rarely eaten. When you do buy it, make sure you purchase the leanest cut available. Before cooking the meat, trim off all visible fat. It's far better to substitute chicken, turkey, and fish. Don't forget to remove that crispy skin off the poultry before eating. Keep your portion size small, 3 ounces is all you really need. You can estimate a portion when eating out—it should be the size of your palm.

Remember beans, grains, and rice are high in protein. Low-fat dairy products are also healthy. But do be careful when purchasing dairy products labeled "low fat." Regular milk contains 3.5 percent fat. Therefore, 2 percent milk, while slightly lower, is not truly low fat. Better to go with skim milk, now called fat free milk, for everything.

CARBOHYDRATES

Start substituting complex carbohydrates (whole grains, breads, pasta, beans, rice, potatoes, and fruits) for sugar. These foods are also rich in fiber, which is important in keeping the bowels regular and preventing colon cancer.

Carbohydrates have had to live with the reputation of being fattening. Now, let the truth be known. Carbohydrates, gram for gram, have the same number of calories as protein (4 calories per gram). Fat, on the other hand, has more than twice that amount (9 calories per gram). Because of this misconception, pasta, potatoes, and other starches are often overlooked when trying to follow a low-calorie diet. This is not to say that sugar can't make you fat. We all know that it can, if eaten in excess. The point is that fat intake presents a greater problem.

Nutritionists recommend that carbohydrates make up 60 percent of our daily caloric intake. Presently, most Americans consume only 45 percent. The bottom line is to dump the fat, while eating more complex carbohydrates.

It is important to understand that not all carbohydrates are created equal. There are three primary groups of carbohydrates. These include refined or simple sugars, starches or complex sugars, and fiber. When nutritionists recommend increasing daily carbohydrate intake, they are referring to starches and fiber. It's not necessary to increase refined sugar, because our bodies can manufacture all the glucose we need from other foods.

Recurrent yeast infections and mood swings can be side effects of consuming excess refined sugar. The first is due to an alteration in vaginal pH. The mood swings occur because the blood sugar is made to rapidly oscillate between very high and very low. With this in mind, remember to reach for fruit instead of candy when you want something sweet.

Complex carbohydrates or starches contain fewer digestible calories. They are also rich in vitamins, minerals, and fiber. All positives with no negatives. How you prepare them is just as important. While it's true that French fries are potatoes, that's not the way to increase your intake of starch. Baked potatoes are far better, but remember to leave off the sour cream and butter. Pasta is the favorite of long distance runners, but sorry, no meat-based gravy.

What is fiber and why is it important? It is a complex carbohydrate which gives structure to fruit, vegetables, and grains. Humans lack the enzymes to digest it, so it travels relatively unchanged through the intestines. It adds bulk which initially satisfies our appetite and later serves to move waste products through the intestines. By increasing the transit of material, it helps to clear potential toxins from the intestines as well. Nitrates from meats are one of these toxins and have been identified as having a causal relationship to colon cancer. Fiber also retains a fair amount of water. This serves to increase the volume and soften the stools, keeping you regular and helping to prevent hemorrhoids. Fiber serves as a natural diuretic and helps to prevent irritable bowel disease. Fiber from oat bran and carrots lowers blood cholesterol and blood sugars levels, providing protection against heart disease and diabetes.

The goal is to eat 20 to 30 grams of fiber a day. Be careful, fiber intake must be increased slowly. A sudden increase can lead to bloating, gas, and diarrhea. Also, drink lots of water. Fiber needs water to move it smoothly through the digestive tract. For this reason, raw fruits and vegetables are good sources of fiber.

FAT

Presently, about 40 percent of the average American dietary calories come from fat. How much do we really need? Only about one tablespoon a day. If you want to lose weight, the only sure way to do it is to drastically reduce your fat intake. Fat, gram for gram, has twice as many calories as carbohydrates and proteins.

We need not cut out all fat from our diet. In fact, we need some for the absorption and storage of fat-soluble vitamins, like A, D, E, and K. Fat is our only source of the essential fatty acid, linolic acid. The nervous system needs linolic acid to function properly, for body temperature regulation, and to help keep our skin smooth and healthy. However, it should not represent more than 30 percent of our daily caloric intake. If you are trying to lose weight, then no more than 15 percent to 20 percent is necessary.

There is another reason for not going "zero fat." When you lower fat intake below a critical level, an interesting phenomenon takes place in your body. It recognizes this as being "fat starved." Any fat that is ingested under these conditions is immediately stored rather than burned. You actually add fat to your body just when you most want to lose it.

Like carbohydrates, not all fats are created equal. There are three types, each differs in how healthy they are for you.

Saturated Fats

Saturated fats are derived from animal products. Tropical oils, solid at room temperature, are the least healthy and should comprise no more than 10 percent of your daily fat.

Monounsaturated Fats

Canola, olive, avocado, and peanut oils are in this group. Canola and olive oil have received attention recently as being helpful in lowering cholesterol. Use them sparingly. They should only represent another 10 percent to 15 percent of daily fat.

Polyunsaturated Fats

The common cooking oils, corn, safflower, sesame, soybean, and sunflower are in this group. Of the three types of fats, these are the least harmful, heartwise. They should comprise 70 percent to 80 percent of our daily fat.

Some foods rich in fat are obvious, such as butter, red meat, and fried foods. However, many times fats can be hidden. We can be eating foods loaded with fat and not even know it. In fact, some of these fats are so well hidden that we may actually think we are eating "health food," only to find out we just consumed a week's worth of fat. Dairy products and nuts are good examples of this. It is because of these hidden fats that we need to become "fat detectives," training ourselves to always be on the lookout for fat. While the National Labeling and Education Act of 1990 made finding fats easier, these labels can sometimes be misleading. A little coaching on how to really interpret the labels is in order.

READ THE LABEL

"Cholesterol free" does not mean "fat free." For example, peanut butter may be labeled cholesterol free but of the 190 total calories per serving, 130 of the calories come from fat. That makes it 70 percent fat! "Lite" also does not mean "fat free" or even "low fat." It means less fat than usually is found in this product. It may still be relatively high in fat content. For example, salad dressings that are 70 calories per serving have 50 calories from fat. Again, 70 percent fat. The calories listed on the label are based on serving size, not the total number of calories per container or box. When was the last time you split a pint of lite ice cream between six people? You must also take serving size into consideration when calculating your calorie consumption.

To calculate the number of calories derived from fat you would multiply the total number of fat grams by 9 calories per gram. To calculate the percent of total calories derived from fat, you would take the calories from fat, divide it by the total calories and then multiply by 100. It is difficult and time consuming to calculate what 30 percent of your total daily calories is going to be (15 percent–20 percent, if trying to lose weight). No one really has that kind of time. As a general rule, try to substitute carbohydrates as much as possible for fats. Look at labels closely, and only eat those fat-containing foods where fat accounts for no more than 15 percent–20 percent of the total calories.

Another example of "unhealthy health foods" are some bran muffins. While usually great sources of fiber, they can also be loaded with fat and refined sugar. If the muffin is heavy and the surface is sticky, it may contain as much butter and sugar as a donut.

Try to get into the habit of baking, oven broiling, and steaming, rather than frying when cooking. Herbs and spices can be used to enhance flavor instead of butter and heavy sauces.

WATER

Comprising 60 percent of a woman's body and 70 percent of a man's, water would appear to be the most important nutrient. Unfortunately, for many of us, it is often the most forgotten nutrient. Outside of being driven by thirst, most of us go through the day oblivious of our water and fluid needs. Water is necessary to transport nutrients, lubricate joints, keep mucous membranes moist, and eliminate water through the urine and bowel.

We require two to three quarts of water each day just to compensate for loses. Half of this water we draw from food sources, such as fruits, vegetables, even bread. The other half comes from the liquids we drink. To remain healthy, we should supplement this with 6 to 8, eight-ounce glasses of either water, juice, or skim milk daily. Caffeinated drinks are poor choices since they also act as diuretics and can lead to an overall loss of water. Soda is also a poor choice since the increased sugar requires a considerable water loss for its excretion in the urine.

MAINTAINING IDEAL WEIGHT

Why do diets often fail, and what can be done to avoid the pitfalls? Most people gain an average of one pound per year after age twenty-five. This occurs not by eating more, but by not eating less. We need to eat less because our metabolism is gradually slowing. This lower metabolism is also the reason why it is much more difficult to lose weight and keep it off in the forties and fifties than it was in the twenties. This translates into an absolute necessity to add exercise to any weight reduction diet. Without exercise, metabolism remains low and reducing calories alone lowers it even further, as the result of a survival reaction.

In order to achieve permanent weight loss, the weight loss must be done gradually. Losing one or two pounds a week may be boring, but it is both healthier and more likely to guarantee long-term success. Radical diets low in calories may initially result in a large weight loss, but unfortunately, most of this weight loss is water loss. Weight loss then plateaus as your body shifts into a "starvation" mode, slowing your metabolism even more. The lack of continued weight loss, coupled with too much denial, dooms the diet to failure. This is sometimes referred to as "yo-yo dieting." You begin a lifetime of repeating the pattern over and over. Even worse, we often gain a few extra pounds with each rebound.

The secret of success, again, is a slow gradual weight loss. This is achieved by balancing the major nutrients, eating smaller portions slowly, and avoiding the pitfalls of denial. It is more appropriate to develop a habit of eating sweets in smaller portions and in moderation. Trying to totally deny ourselves sweets never works. Exercise is also necessary to increase self-esteem. This in turn motivates you to stick with the program.

Surprisingly, a diet rich in complex carbohydrates actually allows you to eat more food. Remember, carbohydrates have only half the calories per gram as fat. Since you can eat more with fewer calories, you seldom feel hungry. Adding something sweet, like fruit not chocolate, at the end of the meal can make you feel satisfied even if your portions of food were smaller.

FAST FACTS
EATING TO STAY FIT

1. *Proteins*
   - ▲ *15 percent total daily caloric intake*
   - ▲ *Get more from vegetables than animal sources*
   - ▲ *Keep meat portions to three ounces.*
   - ▲ *Beans, grains, rice, and low-fat dairy products are good sources.*

2. Carbohydrates

▲ 60 percent total daily caloric intake

▲ Complex carbohydrates are best—whole grain breads, pasta, beans, rice, potatoes, and fruit.

▲ Fiber is important to healthy bowel function and cancer prevention.

3. Fats

▲ 30 percent total caloric intake

▲ 15 percent–20 percent total caloric intake if looking for weight reduction

▲ Fats contain twice as many calories per gram as proteins and carbohydrates.

▲ Eat polyunsaturated and avoid saturated fats.

▲ Limit fat consumption but avoid zero fat diets. This is counterproductive.

▲ Be food label conscious:
  • Check serving size.
  • Calculate the percentage of total calories from fat—number of calories from fat divided by the total calories times 100.

4. Water

▲ Most important nutrient

▲ Supplement with 6 to 8, eight-ounce glasses of water, juice, or skim milk daily.

5. Weight loss is best done slowly and gradually.

6. Other Nutrition Tips

▲ Take a high-potency multivitamin with minerals and iron daily.

▲ Take supplemental calcium.
  • 500 mg if on estrogen replacement or still regularly menstruating
  • 1000 mg if menopausal and not on estrogen replacement
  • Lower sodium intake.
  • Decrease caffeine and use alcohol in moderation.

I

Create Your Own Symptom Diary

Fill out a symptom diary for at least two months and show it to your health care provider.

1. Start the calendar using Day #1 as the first day of your period. Write in the actual month and date.

2. Fill in the calendar dates for the next 30 days.

3. Chart your symptoms daily. Some examples would be:

   ▲ Bleeding

   ▲ Insomnia

   ▲ Headache

EXAMPLE

As you can see from the example on page 89, this woman started her period on April 8th and she bled for four days. She had two days of bleeding on the 14th and 15th days of her cycle, April 21st and April 22nd. On the 18th day, April 25th, she started feeling depressed. This lasted until day 28, May 5th, when her next period started. During this same time, she also experienced insomnia and hot flashes.

SYMPTOM DIARY EXAMPLE

S	M	T	W	T	F	S
1st Day 4/8/98 B	2 4/9/98 B	3 4/10/98 B	4 4/11/98 B	5 4/12/98	6 4/13/98	7 4/14/98
8 4/15/98	9 4/16/98	10 4/17/98	11 4/18/98	12 4/19/98	13 4/20/98	14 4/21/98 B
15 4/22/98 B	16 4/23/98	17 4/24/98	18 4/25/98 D H/S	19 4/26/98 D H/S	20 4/27/98 D H/S	21 4/28/98 D H/S
22 4/29/98 D H/S	23 4/30/98 D H/S	24 5/1/98 D H/S	25 5/2/98 D H/S	26 5/3/98 D H/S	27 5/4/98 D H/S	28 5/5/98 B
29 5/6/98	30 5/7/98	31 5/8/98				

B	=	Bleeding	OK	=	Normal
D	=	Depressed	I	=	Irritable
A	=	Anxious	S	=	Sleep Disturbance
H	=	Hot Flash	*	=	Headache

SYMPTOM DIARY

SYMPTOM DIARY

S	M	T	W	T	F	S

B	=	Bleeding	OK	=	Normal
D	=	Depressed	I	=	Irritable
A	=	Anxious	S	=	Sleep Disturbance
H	=	Hot Flash	*	=	Headache

Asking the
Right Questions

The purpose of this appendix is to prepare you for your appointment with your health care provider in order to discuss your perimenopausal symptoms. Having studied the text of this book, you can now draw on your knowledge in formulating the program best suited to your needs.

Please take some time and fill in the answers to the following questions. They have been presented in the sequence that I have found, as a physician, to be most useful. You will also want to bring copies of your symptom calendars from the past two months to the appointment.

S Y M P T O M S

1. *Referring to your symptom calendars, list the symptoms you have been experiencing, in the order of their severity. For example: Hot flashes, irregular bleeding, etc.*

   1. _____

   2. _____

   3. _____

   4. _____

   5. _____

   6. _____

2. *Menstrual History*

   • How old were you when your periods began? _____

   • Are they regular or irregular? _____

   • How many days between menses? _____

   • Do you experience cramping with your periods? _____
     If yes, grade them from 1 (mild) to 5 (severe). _____

   • Has your flow lightened or increased? _____
     If increased, describe the changes. _____
     _____
     _____

3. *Pregnancy History*

   • How many times were you pregnant? Include miscarriages and terminations. _____
     _____
     _____

   • Did you have vaginal births? _____
     _____
     C Sections? _____
     _____

   • Any complications with pregnancy or delivery? For example: Toxemia, diabetes, hemorrhage after delivery, infection.
     _____
     _____
     _____

4. General Medical Information

- List any medication allergies. _____
  _____
  _____
  _____

- Are you presently taking regular medications, prescription and/or over the counter? _____
  _____
  _____
  _____

- Do you take vitamin, mineral, herbal supplements? If so, which ones? _____
  _____
  _____
  _____

5. Past Medical History

- List any medical conditions you may have. For example: Asthma, thyroid disorder, heart disease, etc. _____
  _____
  _____

- Have you had any surgery? Please list all including childhood surgeries, such as a tonsillectomy. _____
  _____
  _____

- Have you ever had a mammogram? _____
  When was the last study performed? _____
  Was it normal? _____
  If no, explain. _____
  _____
  _____

- When was your last PAP smear? _____
  Was it normal? _____
  If not, explain. _____
  _____
  _____

- Have you ever had a DEXA bone density scan, a Dpd urine test, or a NTx urine test (n-Telopeptide)? _____
  When? _____
  Was it normal? _____
  If no, explain. _____
  _____
  _____

- Have you had your cholesterol/lipid profile checked? _____
  When? _____
  What were the results? _____
  _____
  _____

- Do you smoke? _____
  If yes, how much per day? _____

- How much alcohol do you consume?
  Per Day _____
  Per Month _____
  Other _____
  _____

6. *Family Medical History*

   Please mark all positives. State whether you/family members had the condition.

	YES?	FAMILY
High blood pressure	____	_____
Diabetes	____	_____
Heart problems	____	_____
Stroke	____	_____
Osteoporosis	____	_____
Breast cancer	____	_____
Uterine cancer	____	_____
Cervical cancer	____	_____
Ovarian cancer	____	_____
Colon cancer	____	_____

7. Review of Other Systems

In addition to the symptoms from your calendars, mark any additional problems.

Urinary:

- Loss of urine when you cough, sneeze, or exercise? _____

  _____

  If yes, describe how often, how much, do you need to wear a pad or an adult diaper-type product? _____

  _____

  _____

- Frequent urination? _____

  _____

- Burning with urination? _____

  _____

- Blood in your urine? _____

  _____

Muscles and Joints:

- Arthritis? _____

  _____

- Backache? _____

  _____

- Swelling of ankles or legs? _____

  _____

- Varicose veins? _____

  _____

Stomach and Bowels:

- Abdominal bloating? _____

  _____

- Indigestion? _____

  _____

- Diarrhea/constipation? _____

  _____

S Y M P T O M S

S Y M P T O M S

- Black pasty stools? _____
  _____

- Pencil-like stools? _____
  _____

- Rectal bleeding? _____
  _____

- Abdominal pain not associated with your period? _____
  _____

Lungs and Heart:

- Chest pain? _____
  _____

- Shortness of breath? _____
  _____

- Chronic cough? _____
  _____

- Frequent bloody noses? _____
  _____

Gynecologic:

- Vaginal discharge/odor? _____
  _____

- Vaginal irritation? _____
  _____

- Vulva/vaginal sores or breaks in skin? _____
  _____

- Breast soreness? _____
  _____

- Breast lumps? _____
  _____

- Nipple discharge? _____
  _____

  Color? _____
  _____

- Pelvic pain? _____
  _____

- Painful intercourse? _____
  _____

8. *General:*

- Headaches/migraines? _____
  _____

- Depression? _____
  _____

- Anxiety/irritability? _____
  _____

- Dramatic mood swings? _____
  _____

9. *List your primary physical concerns.*

_____
_____
_____
_____
_____

10. *List your primary emotional concerns.*

_____
_____
_____
_____
_____

11. *Questions for the health care provider to answer.*

- Given my family and personal history, what are my risks of:
  Heart disease? _____
  Osteoporosis? _____
  Breast cancer? _____

- Do these personal risks balance risks and benefits of hormone
  replacement therapy? Why or why not? _____
  _____

S
Y
M
P
T
O
M
S

- If I am only at higher risk for osteoporosis, would it be better for me to follow DEXA scans and start a nonhormonal medication, such as alendonate, if indicated? _____

  _____
  _____
  _____

- If we decide on hormone replacement therapy, which is better for me?

  Continuous _____ Why? _____

  Cyclic _____ Why? _____

  Pills _____ Why? _____

  Patches _____ Why? _____

  What is the name of my medication? Dose?

  Estrogen _____

  _____

  Progestin _____

  _____

- Have any of your patients used nonhormonal treatments for their hot flashes and vaginal dryness? _____

  _____
  _____
  _____

- What worked best for them? _____

  _____
  _____
  _____

- Do you know what health food store or herbalist they used?

  _____
  _____
  _____

Check it Out

1. Pelvic exam
▲ Yearly

2. PAP smear
▲ Yearly

3. Breast exam
▲ Breast self-exam
 – Monthly
 – Perform a week after menses; the first day of each month if no longer menstruating.
▲ Health care provider breast exam
 – Yearly

4. Mammograms
▲ Between age 35 and 40
 – Baseline mammogram should be taken.
▲ Starting at age 40
 – Have mammogram taken every other year after this age.
▲ Starting at age 50
 – Have mammogram taken every year after this age.

5. Laboratory tests
▲ FSH test
 – Test given to determine if starting perimenopause
▲ Fasting lipid profile tests for cholesterol
 – Yearly
▲ Stool check for hidden(occult) blood
 – Yearly
▲ DEXA scan or urine test for bone density
 – Baseline scan between age 45 to 50

SYMPTOM DIARY

S	M	T	W	T	F	S

B	=	Bleeding	OK	=	Normal
D	=	Depressed	I	=	Irritable
A	=	Anxious	S	=	Sleep Disturbance
H	=	Hot Flash	*	=	Headache

SYMPTOM DIARY

S	M	T	W	T	F	S

B	=	Bleeding	OK	=	Normal
D	=	Depressed	I	=	Irritable
A	=	Anxious	S	=	Sleep Disturbance
H	=	Hot Flash	*	=	Headache

SYMPTOM DIARY

S	M	T	W	T	F	S

B	=	Bleeding	OK	=	Normal
D	=	Depressed	I	=	Irritable
A	=	Anxious	S	=	Sleep Disturbance
H	=	Hot Flash	*	=	Headache

SYMPTOM DIARY

S	M	T	W	T	F	S

B	=	Bleeding	OK	=	Normal
D	=	Depressed	I	=	Irritable
A	=	Anxious	S	=	Sleep Disturbance
H	=	Hot Flash	*	=	Headache

S Y M P T O M D I A R Y

S Y M P T O M   D I A R Y

SYMPTOM DIARY

S	M	T	W	T	F	S

B	=	Bleeding	OK	=	Normal
D	=	Depressed	I	=	Irritable
A	=	Anxious	S	=	Sleep Disturbance
H	=	Hot Flash	*	=	Headache

SYMPTOM DIARY

S	M	T	W	T	F	S

B	=	Bleeding	OK	=	Normal
D	=	Depressed	I	=	Irritable
A	=	Anxious	S	=	Sleep Disturbance
H	=	Hot Flash	*	=	Headache

Index

C

Caffeine, avoiding, 50, 67, 77, 85
Calcium carbonate, 18, 40
Calcium loss, diet affecting, 81
Calcium supplements, for reducing hot flashes, 40
Calcium supplements, for reducing osteoporosis risk, 18, 67
Calcium supplements, for reducing PMS, 50
Cancer, *see also specific cancer types*
Cancer, confused with depression, 52
Cancer, estrogen effect on, 26, 28, 58
Cancer, progestin effect on, 30
Carbohydrates, 81-83, 86
Cardiac stress test, 69
Cardiovascular disease, 15
Cardiovascular disease, exercise affecting, 38, 66, 68, 69
Cardiovascular disease, and herbal preparations, 42
Cardiovascular disease, relation to estrogen, 12, 20-21, 25, 26, 31
Cardiovascular disease, relation to testosterone, 59
Cardiovascular disease, risk reduction for, 19, 82
Cardiovascular disease, and vitamin E, 39
Caucasians, cardiovascular disease risk among, 21
Caucasians, osteoporosis risk among, 16
Cervical cap, 61. *see also* Birth control
Chasteberry (*Vitex agnus-castus*), 42
Chills, 60
Chocolate, avoiding, 50
Cholesterol, exercise affecting, 38, 66
Cholesterol, HDL/LDL levels, 20-21, 59
Cholesterol, metabolism of, 20
Cholesterol, reducing, 82, 84
Cholesterol/Lipoprotein profile, reference numbers for, 21
Circulation, enhancement of, 68, 72
Coach, for stress reduction, 51
Colon cancer, 81, 82. *see also* Cancer
Concentration difficulties, due to sleep disturbance, 13
Concentration difficulties, exercise affecting, 66
Concentration difficulties, relation to depression, 51
Condoms, 61. *see also* Birth control
Constipation, due to medications, 19
Coping mechanisms, factors affecting, 49
Counseling, for sexual understanding, 54
Counseling, for stress reduction, 51

Cramping. *see* Leg cramps; Menstrual cramps
Cramps, due to natural progesterone, 44
Cross-country skiing, 67, 73. *see also* Exercise
Cultural attitude, affect on symptoms, 6, 36

D

Dairy products, 15, 40, 81, 84
Deaths, due to osteoporosis, 16
Deaths, from cardiovascular disease, 15
Denial, dietary, 80, 86
Depression, due to natural progesterone, 44
Depression, due to sleep disturbance, 13
Depression, perimenopausal, 48
Depression, symptoms and treatment for, 51-52, 59, 66
DEXA scan, for diagnosing osteoporosis, 17
Diabetes, confused with depression, 52
Diabetes, exercise cautions with, 69
Diabetes, prevention and control of, 68
Diabetes, relation to heart disease, 21
Diabetes, and vitamin E, 39
Diaphragm, 61. *see also* Birth control
Diarrhea, diet affecting, 82
Diarrhea, due to medications, 19
Diet, affect on hot flashes, 38-39
Diet, healthy habits for, 80-87
Diet, label information about, 84-85
Digitalis, and vitamin E, 39
Dioxgenin, 43
Dong quai (*Angelica sinensis*), benefits of, 41
Dpd test, for diagnosing osteoporosis, 17
Drug therapy, confused with depression, 52

E

Early onset menopause, relation to osteoporosis risk, 18
Eating disorders, relation to depression, 51
Echocardiogram, 69
Elders, respect for, 6, 36-37
Emotions. *see* Depression; Moodiness
Empty nest, pros and cons of, 49, 54
Endometrial cancer. *see* Uterine cancer
Endorphins, *see also* Exercise
Endorphins, production and function of, 37, 50, 66
Energy levels, exercise affecting, 38, 66
Energy levels, relation to depression, 51
Estrogen, in birth control pills, 60
Estrogen, combined with progestin, 28-30
Estrogen, effect on breast cancer, 25, 31-33, 40
Estrogen, "endogenous", 29, 66-67
Estrogen, from plants, 38-39

Estrogen, ratio to testosterone, 54
Estrogen, role in menstrual cycle, 8, 10
Estrogen, types of, "designer estrogens", 27-28
Estrogen, types of, estradiol, 26
Estrogen, types of, estriol 26
Estrogen, types of, estrone, 26
Estrogen, types of, triple estrogen ("triest"), 27
Estrogen, vaginal cream, 30-31, 55, 56-57
Estrogen loss effects, 12-23. *see also*
      Hormone replacement therapy
Estrogen loss effects, cardiovascular disease,
      20-21
Estrogen loss effects, emotional changes, 15
Estrogen loss effects, hot flashes, 12-13, 37
Estrogen loss effects, mental effects, 13
Estrogen loss effects, osteoporosis, 12,
      15-19, 24-25
Estrogen loss effects, vaginal effects, 13-14, 15
Exercise, aerobic, 69, 70-71, 73
Exercise, benefits of, 38, 50, 66, 85
Exercise, confused with activity level, 68-69
Exercise, cross-country skiing, 67, 73
Exercise, "cross-training", 71
Exercise, effect on endorphins, 37, 50
Exercise, effect on hot flashes, 37-38
Exercise, friends for, 77
Exercise, Kegel exercises, 14
Exercise, metabolic changes with, 68-69, 85-86
Exercise, personal trainers for, 76
Exercise, program design for, 69-70
Exercise, progress recordkeeping for, 76
Exercise, recommendations for, 67-74
Exercise, for reducing heart disease risk, 21
Exercise, for reducing osteoporosis risk, 18
Exercise, sample schedule for, 76
Exercise, scientific background for, 66-67
Exercise, stretching, 69, 74-76
Exercise, water aerobics, 18
Exercise, weight training, 69, 73-74

F

Family history, relation to heart disease, 21
Family history, relation to osteoporosis risk,
      17-18
Fat, monounsaturated, 83
Fat, polyunsaturated, 84
Fat, reducing in diet, 81, 83
Fat, saturated, 83
Fat, unsaturated, 40
Fat metabolism, estrogen affect on, 20
Fatigue, due to natural progesterone, 44
Fatigue, pre-menstrual, 49
Fennel tea, benefits of, 39
Fever, 60

Fiber, role in diet, 81, 82-83
Fluid retention, *see also* Water
Fluid retention, estrogen affecting, 25, 29
Fluid retention, reducing, 50
Foam, 61. *see also* Birth control
Follicle stimulating hormone (FSH), role in
      menstrual cycle, 8, 10
Forgetfulness, due to sleep disturbance, 13
FSH. *see* Follicle stimulating hormone`

G

Gallbladder disease, 40
Ginseng (*Panax ginseng*), 42

H

Headache, due to natural progesterone, 44
Headache, estrogen affecting, 25
Health, diet affecting, 80-87
Health care provider, information available
      from, 25, 28, 69
Heart disease. *see* Cardiovascular disease
Heartburn, due to medications, 19
Herbs, as calcium supplements, 40
Herbs, for symptom reduction, 40-43
Hip fracture, due to osteoporosis, 16
Hormone replacement therapy (HRT), *see
      also* Estrogen; Progestin; Testosterone
Hormone replacement therapy (HRT),
      allergic response to, 30, 31
Hormone replacement therapy (HRT), cal-
      cium supplements combined with, 18
Hormone replacement therapy (HRT),
      cyclic or continuous use, 29
Hormone replacement therapy (HRT), goal
      of, 25-26
Hormone replacement therapy (HRT), nat-
      ural estrogen combination pill, 26
Hormone replacement therapy (HRT),
      patches vs. pills, 28, 29, 30, 31
Hormone replacement therapy (HRT), rec-
      ommendations for, 5, 19, 24-25
Hormone replacement therapy (HRT),
      vaginal estrogen cream, 30-31, 55, 56-57
Hormone replacement therapy (HRT),
      withdrawal symptoms, 25
Hot flashes, diet affecting, 38-39
Hot flashes, discussion of, 12-13, 36-37
Hot flashes, estrogen loss affecting, 12-13,
      37, 60, 67
Hot flashes, exercise affecting, 37-38
Hot flashes, herbal remedies for, 41-42
Hot flashes, natural progesterone for, 43-44
Hot flashes, supplements affecting, 39-40
HRT. *see* Hormone replacement therapy

Human Chorionic Gonadotropin (HCG), role in menstrual cycle, 8
Hypertension, *see also* Blood pressure
Hypertension, exercise cautions with, 69
Hypertension, herbal remedies cautions with, 42, 43
Hypertension, relation to heart disease, 21
Hypertension, and vitamin E, 39
Hypothalamus, 37
Hysterectomy, estrogen recommendations with, 28, 30

I

Impotence, 57
In-vitro fertilization (IVF), 62
Infection, confused with depression, 52
Infection, vaginal, 55
Insomnia, *see also* Sleep disturbance
Insomnia, pre-menstrual, 49
Insomnia, relation to estrogen loss, 12
Intestinal gas, diet affecting, 82
Intestinal gas, due to calcium supplements, 18
Intestinal gas, due to medications, 19
Intestinal upset, *see also* Bloating; Stomach disorder
Intestinal upset, estrogen recommendations with, 28
Intrauterine device (IUD), *see also* Birth control
Intrauterine device (IUD), recommendations for, 60
"Involutional Melancholia", 48
Iron supplements, 50
Irritability, pre-menstrual, 49, 50
Irritable bowel disease, 82
IUD. *see* Intrauterine device
IVF. *see* In-vitro fertilization

J

Joint pain/inflammation, exercise recommendations for, 18

K

Kegel exercises, discussion of, 14
Kidney disease, herbal remedies cautions with, 43
Kinsey report, 54

L

Lee, John R., M.D., 27
Leg cramps, estrogen affecting, 25
LH. *see* Luteinizing Hormone
Libido, exercise affecting, 68

Libido, hormonal basis for, 54, 57, 59
Licorice root (*Glycyrrhiza glabra*), 43
Lifestyle modification, for stress reduction, 50
Linolic acid, 83
Liver disease, estrogen recommendations with, 28
Liver disease, testosterone effect on, 58, 59
Longevity, relation to osteoporosis, 15
Luteinizing Hormone (LH), role in menstrual cycle, 8

M

Mammograms, 33. *see also* Breast cancer
Marker, Dr. Russell, 43
Masculinizing effects, *see also* Libido
Masculinizing effects, from testosterone application, 59
Masters and Johnson report, 54
Mayan Indians, menopausal symptoms in, 36-37
Meat, 81, 82. *see also* Diet
Men, sexual function in, 57
Menopause, *see also* Perimenopause
Menopause, birth control pills affecting, 60
Menopause, surgical, 58
Menstrual cramps, herbal remedies for, 40, 41
Menstrual cycle, 7. *see also* Birth control; Bleeding
Menstrual cycle, follicular phase, 8
Menstrual cycle, with hormone replacement therapy, 29
Menstrual cycle, luteal phase, 8
Menstrual cycle, ovulatory phase, 8
Menstrual cycle, pre-menopause irregularity in, 10-11
Menstrual cycle, as signal for breast exam, 33
Mental effects, due to estrogen loss, 13
Metabolic change, exercise affecting, 68-69
Metabolism, of fat, 20
Methyltestosterone, *see also* Testosterone
Methyltestosterone, advantages and disadvantages, 58
Moodiness, *see also* Depression; Pre-menstrual syndrome
Moodiness, diet affecting, 82
Moodiness, due to sleep disturbance, 13, 15
Moodiness, exercise affecting, 66

N

Nausea, due to medications, 19
Norethindrone, 43
NTx test, for diagnosing osteoporosis, 17
Nurses Health Study, 31-32, 68

O

P

R

S

Smoking, relation to osteoporosis risk, 18

Soy products, phytoestrogens in, 39

Spinal deformity, due to osteoporosis, 16

Sterilization, 61. *see also* Birth control

Stomach disorder, *see also* Bloating; Intestinal upset

Stomach disorder, due to medications, 19

Stomach disorder, estrogen affecting, 25, 30

Stress, perimenopausal, 48, 49

Stress, relation to heart disease, 21

Stress reduction, with exercise, 38, 50, 67, 68, 72

Stress reduction, recommendations for, 50-51

Stretching, 69, 74-76. *see also* Exercise

Sugar, avoiding, 50, 67, 81, 82, 85

Suicide, 51

Supplements, affect on hot flashes, 39-40

Swimming, 18, 67, 72. *see also* Exercise

Symptoms, attitude affecting, 6

Symptoms journal, 49-50

T

Tai Chi, 75

Testosterone, *see also* Hormone replacement therapy

Testosterone, considerations for using, 57-59

Testosterone, methyltestosterone{,} advantages and disadvantages, 58

Testosterone, natural, 58-59

Testosterone, role in sex drive, 54

Tests, for cholesterol, 20

Tests, for osteoporosis, 16-19

Thyroid disorder, confused with depression, 52

Treadmill, 18

Tubal ligation, 61-62. *see also* Birth control

U

Urethra, estrogen loss affecting, 13-14, 30

Urinary tract disorder, diaphragm use affecting, 61

Urinary tract disorder, herbal remedies cautions with, 43

Urinary tract disorder, misdiagnosis of, 13

Urination, burning and incontinence with, 13, 14, 30

Urine test, for diagnosing osteoporosis, 17

Uterine cancer, *see also* Cancer

Uterine cancer, birth control choices affecting, 60

Uterine cancer, estrogen effect on, 32, 40

Uterine cancer, progestin effect on, 30

Uterus, progestin affect on, 30

V

Vagina, estrogen creme for, 30-31

Vagina, estrogen/progestin insertion in, 30

Vagina, lubrication recommendations for, 55, 56

Vaginal cream, *see also* Estrogen

Vaginal cream, recommendations for, 30-31, 55, 56-57

Vaginal dryness, diet affecting, 38-39

Vaginal dryness, estrogen loss affecting, 12, 15, 30, 31, 677

Vaginal dryness, herbal remedies for, 42

Vaginal dryness, moisturizers for, 55-56

Vaginal dryness, natural progesterone for, 43-44

Vaginal dryness, sexual activity affecting, 56

Vaginal effects, due to estrogen loss, 12, 13-14, 15, 55

Vasectomy, 61. *see also* Birth control

Vegetables, 40, 81

Vision impairment, 40

Vitamin B-complex, 40, 50, 67

Vitamin C, 40, 67

Vitamin E, 39, 50, 56

Vulva, physical changes in, 15, 55

Vulva, testosterone application to, 59

W

Walking, 67, 72. *see also* Exercise

Water, *see also* Fluid retention

Water, in diet, 82-83, 85

Weight, *see also* Obesity; Overweight

Weight, ideal maintenance, 85-86

Weight, relation to osteoporosis risk, 17-18

Weight training, 69, 70, 73-74. *see also* Exercise

Western culture, perimenopause attitude in, 6, 36

Western Washington State Study, 32

Wild yam (*Dioscorea villosa*), natural estrogen from, 27

Wild yam (*Dioscorea villosa*), natural progesterone from, 43-44

Wrinkles, reduction of, 68

Y

Yeast infection, diet affecting, 82

Yeast infection, misdiagnosis of, 13

Yoga, 51, 75

Other books in the Vital Information Series

Surgery

By Molly Shapiro, M.B.A., R.N.

So, you may be facing surgery. Whether this is your first surgery or not, health care is different today. Surgery covers every aspect of the surgery process including what your rights are as a patient. It tells you how to prepare for surgery, what happens in surgery, explains equipment use and procedures, and answers your post-op concerns.

$11.95 • ISBN 0-89594-898-2

Hospitals

By Diane Barnet, M.S., R.N.

Hospitals can be intimidating places. Many consumers don't know how to obtain information or even what questions to ask. *Hospitals* provides inside information for patients and their advocates. It explains how hospitals function, and includes an overview of our body systems and a user-friendly guide to medical equipment, procedures, and drugs.

$11.95 • ISBN 0-89594-908-3

Vitamins, Minerals & Supplements

By Gayle Skowronski and Beth Petro Roybal

Vitamins, Minerals & Supplements gives information about the role of supplements in nutrition and how to choose them wisely. It gives details for specific common nutritional supplements and the daily requirements necessary to maintain good health plus a cross-referenced list by ailment.

$11.95 • ISBN 0-89594-935-0

To receive a current catalog from The Crossing Press,
please call toll-free,
800-777-1048.
Visit our Website on the Internet at: www.crossingpress.com